U.S.A.'s
#1
HEALTH
PRIORITY

A.I.D.S.

EVERYTHING YOU MUST KNOW ABOUT

BY
JANET
BAKER

Acquired Immune Deficiency Syndrome

THE KILLER EPIDEMIC OF THE 80'S

FOREWORD BY SANDY POMERANTZ, M.D.

DEDICATION BY HARVEY THOMPSON, M.D.

Published by
R & E Publishers
P. O. Box 2008
Saratoga, California 95070
Robert D. Reed, Publisher

I.S.B.N. 0-88247-700-5

PUBLISHER'S THANKS

To put a book out in ten days takes many talented and dedicated people. We saw the need for an informative overview of the A.I.D.S. epidemic and had the help of many. The people listed below get the credit for a job well done.

TYPOGRAPHY — ESTELLA KREBS
COVER TYPE — DUO TYPE, PALO ALTO, CALIFORNIA
COVER PRINTING — MOODY PRINTING, MT. VIEW, CALIFORNIA
PUBLICITY — HARRY REED

TABLE OF CONTENTS

LIST OF TABLES

LIST OF ILLUSTRATIONS

DEDICATION

There has never been such a health problem as A.I.D.S.

A.I.D.S. is the worst possible scenario of an Andromeda strain come true. It is a disease that looks to be 100% lethal, has no known cause, no known test and no known cure.

A.I.D.S. rocks the very foundations of the gay and lesbian community. It will forever alter how they relate to one another, where they live, how they live and even IF they live. It will also change the way society relates to them and, in turn, have an effect on the straight community, even the price of real estate.

All too often, the person with a disease is forgotten; attention instead is given to the disease's medical aspects. An example of this was the recent second National A.I.D.S. Forum in Denver, Colorado, mid-June 1983.

The last morning had been one dull report after another. The audience had forgotten that A.I.D.S. is not just crisis centers, information pamphlets, T-cell ratios and hot-lines but, instead, A.I.D.S. is also people.

Experts had gathered from across the nation and over 300 people attended. But everyone was upstaged by the nine "People with A.I.D.S." who closed the session with their own "statement."

When they entered the room and walked down the aisle, there was, at first, just a ripple of applause; it rose and crested to a tidal wave by the time they assembled at the front. When they unfurled the banner that read, "WE ARE FIGHTING FOR OUR LIVES," the audience was on its feet.

They preferred not being called victims for that implied hopelessness. They perferred not to be called patients for that implied passivity.

Instead, they looked confident — not ashamed. They looked as if they knew something of life that we didn't, or possibly they knew something of death that we didn't. Dying seems a topic even more taboo in America than is talk of homosexuality.

These were the people who had their numbers drawn in the giant A.I.D.S. lottery. They didn't look like drug-abusers, or fisters, or bath-dwellers. Some were gaunt, some were bald and some were strikingly handsome. They were all about the same age; for sure, they were too young to die.

Irrational fears surfaced when one of the nine people with A.I.D.S. brushed an elbow on the way down the aisle. You recognized another as one who had used the same sweaty sit-up board in the hotel gym the day before. You caught a glimpse of the public hysteria in yourself. Just a few days before, the whole conference had almost aborted when the hotel management objected to the use of the word "A.I.D.S." on lobby posters.

Then the nine men began their roll call and each name brought a shudder of relief when it wasn't yours, and you thought to yourself: OH MY GOD, it's true; there are hundreds of us dying. Then the fear turned to anger and you shouted to yourself: Why doesn't someone DO SOMETHING!

The nine people with A.I.D.S. took turns reading off their rights: to full and satisfying sexual, emotional lives, to quality medical care, to full explanations and the right to refuse treatment or research, to privacy and, lastly, to live and die in dignity.

They asked for support in the struggle against those who could fire them, evict them from their jobs, refuse to touch them or treat them. They asked for support in not losing their loved ones or becoming the scapegoats for an epidemic.

To the health-care providers, they asked that we 'come-out' to them. That we too get in touch with our feelings about A.I.D.S. and examine our own agendas. They wanted to be dealt with not just intellectually but as whole people with complex social needs as well as medical.

They, in turn, promised to try to become involved in every level of decision-making, to share their experiences and knowledge, and to inform any potential partner of their health status, and to substitute low-risk sexual behavior.

One of the people with A.I.D.S. asked the audience to close their eyes. Then he asked us to hold the hand of the person next to us. He began his slow, prepared narrative. . .

He spoke of love and asked us to concentrate on it radiating out to the people with A.I.D.S.: to the already-dead and to the soon-to-die. His voice cracked, wavered and halted. Each time we wondered if he could go on then but there would be a dry-mouthed swallow and a quick nasal inspiratory sniffle of recovery to clear the tears before they fell.

He asked that we recognize that quality is better than quantity, that dying is a part of living and that we come to grips with our own mortality. And the love grew; it filled the room. I expected a miracle: the purple spots would disappear, hair would grow back and flesh fill out again. I wouldn't even now be surprised to hear it happened.

We were told to hug the person next to us and our spirits joined together. We envisioned the love and energy soaring out of the hotel and into the Rockies. It spilled down the sunny slopes into the streets of both coasts. It overflowed up the stairs and down the hallways into gay households all across America that only this kind of brotherly love could enfold.

The tension broke into the relief of tears and we held the whole gay and lesbian community in our arms; laughing and crying, crying and laughing.

I hope those nine men draw on that love when they need it. I hope that if they close their eyes for a last time sometime soon, some of their thoughts will be of us and how we loved 'em in Denver. I'll never forget. To them this space is dedicated.

Harvey Thompson, M.D.
Co-Medical Director
Kaposi's Sarcoma Foundation
Sacramento, California
June 16, 1983

FOREWORD

A.I.D.S.—Acquired Immune Deficiency Syndrome, initially termed Gay-Related Immunodeficiency State, reared its ugly head in mid-1981 when the first cases of Kaposi's sarcoma (KS) and subsequently pneumocystis carinii pneumonia (PCP) were first reported. Since that time, over 1600 persons have been identified with A.I.D.S., and over 600 people have now died from this set of disorders which have been so clearly defined in the ensuing pages. Why? Well, that still remains shrouded in medical mystery. Nevertheless, one thing is clear. The problem is a fundamental defect in the immune system which has permitted the "opportunity" of a variety of viral, fungal, parasitic and bacterial infections to occur, as well as three forms of cancer—Kaposi's sarcoma, non-Hodgkins' lymphoma and anorectal carcinoma.

Janet Baker has compiled a rather extensive chronology of the understanding of A.I.D.S. and its impact, particularly amongst Gay men. While the understanding about A.I.D.S. and the A.I.D.S. disorders continues to evolve and change, the presentation done by Ms. Baker well documents the chronology of events and presents in an understandable way the current speculations about etiology, transmissibility, present treatment regimens; it also points to the possible horizons about each.

This is the dissemination of non-sensational information about the A.I.D.S.-related disorders and their effect(s) on those who are at highest risk for their occurrence. These groups include sexually active, multi-partnered Gay men, natives of Haiti, IV drug abusers, patients with hemophilia, the sexual partners of those groups, the offspring of these high-risk parents and some speculative data on persons who have received blood transfusions.

The objectives have been achieved, with careful documentations, using sources that are well respected within the scientific and Gay communities. False leads and misconceptions will only be recognized with hindsight as the epidemic unfolds. For example, what was at first thought to be an epidemic of cancer instead turned out to be an epidemic of immune deficiency. Also, amyl nitrate, at first thought to be a strong etiological suspect, is now low on the list as other population groups became involved.

Janet Baker compiled parts of this text as a university project. She is married and the mother of two college-age sons. Her heterosexual viewpoint is an advantage for objectivity. To quote an oft-used phrase, it is sometimes easier to see the forest when you are not among the trees.

It is, therefore, with pleasure that I highly recommend this book to all who are concerned about this Number 1 public health hazard of the 80's — to the general public as well as to any person in a high risk category.

Sandy Pomerantz, M.D.
Co-Medical Director
Sacramento A.I.D.S./KS Foundation

PREFACE

The most difficult aspect of A.I.D.S. is its definition. Taken word-by-word, A.I.D.S. is: 1) Acquired, 2) A deficient immune system, and 3) A syndrome with a variety of manifestations.

The stricter definition is the one now used by the U. S. Center for Disease Control as outlined in the Morbidity and Mortality Weekly Report, September 24, 1982, Volume 31, No. 37. CDC defines a case of A.I.D.S. "as a disease, at least moderately predictive of a defect in cell-mediated immunity occurring in a person with no known cause for diminished resistance to that disease."

CDC admits that this case definition may not include the full spectrum of A.I.D.S., which could range from no symptoms (despite laboratory evidence of immune deficiency) to non-specific symptoms (fever, weight-loss, lymphadenopathy—generalized swollen glands). Also, the full spectrum of A.I.D.S. could include diseases that are now thought insufficiently predictive of immunodeficiency such as tuberculosis, oral candidiasis, or herpes zoster. On the other hand, perhaps some patients who have diseases that are only moderately predictive of cellular immunodeficiency may not actually be immunodeficient at all and, therefore, not part of the present epidemic.

Unfortunately, since there is no test presently available that is reliable to make a diagnosis of A.I.D.S., the CDC definition is our most useful tool. It is worth memorizing. Once again, A.I.D.S. is a disease, at least moderately predictive of a defect in a cell-mediated immunity, that occurs in a person with no known cause for diminished resistance to that disease.

It is a difficult diagnosis to make. If there was ever a need for a second medical opinion, this disease is it. The diseases that are moderately predictive of the defect in cell-mediated immunity are not easy to prove. For example, the Kaposi's sarcoma, a cancer that is related to immune deficiency, has difficult histology that can be missed by competent pathologists. Another example is the pneumocystis carinii protozoa that is not easily recovered from the pneumonia patient with A.I.D.S.

Almost to an agent, each infection is not familiar to most physicians. Some of these infections, like cryptosporidiosis, are not even found in standard textbooks. All of the names except herpes are jawbreakers: progressive multifocal leukoencephalopathy, cytomegalovirus, histoplasmosis, cryptococcosis, strongyloidosis, toxoplasmosis, coccidioidomycosis, etc.

When physicians cannot easily understand A.I.D.S. and its manifestations, how then can the general public? The herpes problem is a problem blown out of proportion or at least pales in comparison to A.I.D.S. Yet the public outcry in response to herpes was and continues to be enormous. To ask the public to rationally understand A.I.D.S. is nearly impossible, yet to contain the now growing hysterical response is mandatory.

The most difficult task of all is to ask the patient who is dying with A.I.D.S. to understand. It is this person who must deal with not only this fatal disease, but must also cope with the hysteria, stigmatism, and, in far too many instances, the homophobia (in the case of gay men) spreading throughout the public at large.

    This book will help educate physicians, patients and the general public. It is incomplete, to be sure, but so too is the final story on this, the most tragic and major epidemic of our century.

Sandy Pomerantz, M.D.
Co-Medical Director, A.I.D.S. Clinic
University of California
Davis Medical Center
Sacramento, California

Harvey Thompson, M.D.
Co-Medical Director, A.I.D.S. Clinic
University of California
Davis Medical Center
Sacramento, California

INTRODUCTION

War, famine and pestilence, many times causing one another, have been a menace and curse upon mankind for centuries, with pestilence often being the most destructive and horrifying of them all.

Plagues contributed to the downfall of ancient Rome and Athens. The Black Death wrought disaster upon Europe in the fourteenth century. Venereal disease has claimed millions of victims over the years with devastating consequences. It plagued Henry VIII and possibly contributed to the insanity of Ivan the Terrible. Napoleon's army crumbled in defeat to Russia partially because of a widespread influx of typhus just as the Aztecs were defeated in Mexico after suffering an onslaught of smallpox.

As our civilization seems to move ahead with our advanced knowledge and technology, we continue to be faced with new and unforeseen health threats, some of them without cure. We often seem defenseless in the face of attack from widespread outbreaks of diseases, commonly known as "epidemics."

As Geoffrey Marks and William Beatty, in their book *Epidemics* stated:

"Epidemic diseases have provided some of the most mystifying, exciting and devastating chapters in the history of mankind.

Many definitions of an epidemic exist. I have chosen a fairly loose one: an epidemic is a generally communicable disease that affects many persons at one time. Two major exceptions to this are: a non-communicable disease that affects a large number of individuals in a group or locality (for example, legionnaires disease) and a disease that is remarkable for some specially noticeable or frightening feature but which only affects a relatively small number of people (for example, toxic shock syndrome).

Even in modern times there is still much that we do not know about the causes, spread and decline of many epidemic diseases. Powerful new methods of treatment have sometimes complicated the picture by stimulating the development of resistant microorganisms. Unexplainable appearances of new or mutated strains can burst unexpectedly on an unsuspecting population. Man can even, unfortunately, create an epidemic where none existed before.

The three words that make up the 'demic' family can be thought of, and kept separate in the following terms. An endemic (from the Green 'en' meaning 'on' and 'demos,' 'the people') disease is one that is a part of everyday life in a region. An endemic disease can be likened to the large living room rug that everyone accepts and doesn't bother to think about intil its loose edge trips up occasional visitors. An epidemic ('epi' means 'in') disease can be thought of as being an explosion that affects a large number of people or creates a strikingly noticeable impact. A pandemic ('pan' means 'all') disease is essentially an enlarged epidemic that affects a greater number of people over a broader area. Pandemics may be thought of as chain-reaction explosions."[1]

It is my goal with this book, from a layman's point of view, to explore some facts and hopefully shed some light on a recent and bizarre epidemic that has the potential of sweeping across America, and possibly the world, with devastating and deadly consequences.

According to a statement made by Dr. David Sencer, Commissioner of the New York City Department of Health, in an article published January 31, 1983, in the *New York Native*:

> "A.I.D.S. is perhaps the most serious epidemic of a new infectious
> disease in this country since polio."

A.I.D.S. — THE KILLER EPIDEMIC OF THE 80's

INTRODUCTION FOOTNOTES

[1]Geoffrey Marks and William Beatty, *Epidemics*, (New York: Scribners, 1976), Preface xi, xii.

CHAPTER I
What Is A.I.D.S.?

"Medical detectives are calling it the century's most virulent epidemic. It is as relentless as leukemia, as contagious as hepatitis and its cause has eluded researchers for more than two years. It was first seen in homosexual men — particularly those who were promiscuous — but it has now struck so many different groups that its course cannot be predicted.

Despite a massive nationwide hunt involving hundreds of investigators and millions of dollars, scientists simply cannot catch up with it."[1]

"Acquired immune deficiency syndrome (A.I.D.S.) is the name given to a recently reported complex of health problems. All patients with A.I.D.S. have developed a severe loss of their natural immunity against disease, leaving them vulnerable to illnesses that might not otherwise be a threat. These illnesses are often referred to as opportunistic infections."[2]

Dr. Lawrence Mass, in his article for *New York Native*, states:

"A.I.D.S. is a newly documented and poorly understood disorder in which part of the body's immune system is damaged in varying degrees of severity. As a result, some victims of A.I.D.S. are more vulnerable than others to a growing number of serious, often fatal, diseases.

The two most frequently reported of these diseases continue to be an otherwise rare form of cancer called Kaposi's sarcoma (KS) and a more common protozoan infection of the lungs called pneumocystis carinii pneumonia (PSP) that is not ordinarily seen in immunologically healthy individual."[3]

"The mysterious A.I.D.S. organism is generally thought to be a virus or other infectious agent (as opposed to a bacterium) and to be spread in bodily secretions, especially blood and semen. A.I.D.S. leaves the victim prey to cancers and opportunistic infections that the body is unable to defend against. And, while some of the diseases associated with A.I.D.S. can be successfully treated, the underlying immune problem is, apparently, irreversible. The A.I.D.S. patient may survive his first bizarre infection, or his second, but he remains vulnerable to successive infections, one of which is likely to kill him."[4]

"Kaposi's sarcoma, a cancer, is only one of a dozen serious diseases currently threatening the lives of young men and women worldwide. The diseases are collectively known as acquired immune deficiency syndrome (A.I.D.S.). Diseases such as Kaposi's sarcoma and Pneumocystis carinii pneumonia (PCP) are life-threatening. Others are less so. All appear to be associated with a state of immune deficiency that severely impairs the ability of the body to suppress disease-causing organisms and certain kinds of cancer

1

cells. Following are some of the A.I.D.S. diseases:

1. Cryptococcosis is caused by a fungus that can infect the brain, lungs, liver, intestinal tract and skin of the immunocompromised host.

2. Non-Hodgkins lymphoma is a cancer of the lymph nodes that is now being reported at a greater-than-expected frequency among immunodeficient gay men.

3. Candidiasis is a yeast infection that takes advantage of the immune deficiency state and can cause overwhelming and sometimes difficult to treat infections of the mouth, anus, genitals and other areas of the body.

4. Herpes simplex is a widespread virus that frequently causes localized "fever blisters" or eruptions on the skin of the face, buttocks, anus or genitals. However, in immunodeficient individuals, herpes can produce persistent lesions that cover large areas of the body.

5. CMV is a widespread virus that usually produces symptoms similar to infectious mononucleosis, or may produce no overt symptoms whatsoever. In the immunodeficient individual, CMV can lead to serious and debilitating infections including pneumonia.

5. Toxoplasmosis is a parasitic infection that can involve brain tissues and cause central nervous system disorders in the immunodeficient person. It is usually characterized by severe flu-like symptoms and malaise."[5]

Dr Mass, in his *New York Native* article, goes on to say:

"There are currently at least 22 cases of an uncommon disorder of blood clotting in gay men, some of whom are immunodeficient, in the New York City area. This disorder is called autoimmune thrombocytopenia purpura (ATP). It is not known yet if ATP is part of or otherwise connected to A.I.D.S. But the sudden appearance of this abnormality of immune regulation in the same population, at the same time and in the same principal location as the A.I.D.S. epidemic suggests more than coincidence.

In diseases of autoimmunity, the immune system attacks not only foreign invaders like viruses and bacteria but the actual tissues of the body as well. In ATP, it is the platelets necessary for normal blood clotting that are attacked and injured by the patient's own antibodies. The symptoms of ATP are easy bruisability or unexplained bleeding and may include enlargement of the spleen. The laboratory diagnosis of ATP begins with a complete blood count (CBC) which includes a platelet count. Steroids and sometimes splenectomy (removal of the spleen) have been used to treat ATP. In those patients who also have A.I.D.S, however, the safety of using immunosuppressive steroids is less certain. Some observers feel that plasmapheresis (see Appendix B) holds promise in the treatment of such cases."[6]

According to Susan West, in her article on A.I.D.S. printed in the March 1983 issue of *Science 83* magazine, entitled "One Step Behind a Killer":

"A.I.D.S. has struck 1,200 people as of March 1983 and it has killed 450 of them.* Almost three-fourths of the people who first got the disease are dead. Some researchers believe no one survives it.

2

Since it was detected in 1981, the number of cases has doubled every six months. So far, it has hit young homosexual men, users of intravenous drugs and their sexual partners, Haitians, Hemophiliacs and children. Acquired Immune Deficiency Syndrome: 'acquired' to indicate its victims didn't inherit it, 'immune deficiency' because the one thing they have in common is a breakdown of their immune systems, and 'syndrome' to cover the grab bag of rare but ravaging diseases that take advantage of their bodies' collapsed defenses.

It's the syndrome part that kills them. At first they feel as though they might have the flu, as if they've been to one party too many. But six to 18 months later they still feel that way; they don't know it, but they have lost their ability to fight off disease. Then about a third of them develop Kaposi's sarcoma, Pneumocystis carinii, or any of the arm-long list of so-called opportunistic infections — including rare cancers and diseases caused by fungi, herpes and other viruses, bacteria and protozoans — that don't affect people whose immune systems are working properly. With treatment the victims may overcome one of these only to succumb to another because their natural defenses never seem to rally.

Everything about A.I.D.S. looks as though it is contagious. Scientists think it is passed by 'intimate contact' — shared drug needles, for example, or sexual intercourse. Which points to something carried by the bloodstream. This has a lot of health officials worried about the millions of people who give and receive blood.

The problem is, no one knows a cure. No one even knows the cause.

Before this epidemic, Kaposi's sarcoma and pneumocystis were rare. In the United States, Kaposi's most often shows up in older men of Jewish and Mediterranean descent. It also afflicts males of all ages in Africa, particularly Uganda. It starts as small purplish spots, almost like bruises, usually on the feet and legs. Until the A.I.D.S. epidemic, it was not considered particularly deadly. Physicians were used to encountering pneumocystis as well as Kaposi's in kidney transplant patients whose immune systems are temporarily knocked out so they won't reject the kidney or in cancer victims treated by chemotherapy.

The scientists also knew of conditions that could cripple a person's immune system. Common viral illnesses such as influenza and mononucleosis, for example, cause transient immune deficiencies. So do transfusions and malnutrition. They also knew of the link between viruses and cancer: Viruses cause cancer in animals and a virus has been isolated that is believed to cause a type of human leukemia.

Then they began learning about A.I.D.S. One of the first and most important characteristic they noticed was the peculiar type of immune defect these patients have. Patients with A.I.D.S. have normal or elevated amounts of antibodies and of the cells that make them. But the white blood cells called helper T cells, which assist the antibodies and anti-body-making cells, are very low in number. Moreover, their counterparts, which inhibit the antibody system and are called suppressor T cells, are not affected. With more suppressor cells than helper cells, the immune system is held back from attacking foreign organisms."[7]

"While immune-function tests that measure the ratio of T cells are available, most doctors and clinicians advise people at risk for A.I.D.S. against having them. The tests are expensive, ranging from $100 to $600, and the results are virtually impossible to interpret with any accuracy.

Many people show signs of 'lymphadenopathy syndrome' — they have chronically swollen glands and damaged immune function. Doctors do not know if this is a passing condition, a mild form of A.I.D.S. or a harbinger of worse to come. All they know is that immune abnormalities have been found in as many as 80 percent of the homosexual men in New York City whose T-cell ratios were measured, even though most of them were apparently healthy. But no one ever looked for immune-function problems in these individuals before, so it is not clear what the findings mean. Investigators have embarked on some long-term studies to follow what happens to these men."[8]

West further states in her article in *Science 83*:

"Much of the evidence that epidemiologists have turned up seems to indicate that something like a virus is causing A.I.D.S."[9]

CHAPTER I FOOTNOTES

[1]Robin Marantz Henig, "AIDS — A New Disease's Deadly Odyssey," *New York Times Magazine*, (6 February 1983), p. 28.

[2]U. S. Department of Health and Human Services, Public Health Service, Centers for Disease Control, *"Questions and Answers On Acquired Immune Deficiency Syndrome (A.I.D.S.)"* November 1982.

[3]Lawrence Mass, M.D., "Basic Questions, Basic Answers About The Epidemic," *New York Native*, III, no. 3, (3-16 January 1983),p. 21.

[4]Henig, *New York Times Magazine*.

[5]Kaposi's Sarcoma Foundation. *"Kaposi's Sarcoma and Other Diseases of the Acquired Immune Deficiency Syndrome,"* San Francisco.

[6]Mass, "Basic Questions," *New York Native*.

[7]Susan West, "One Step Behind A Killer," *Science 83*, IV, No. 2, (March 1983), p. 37.

*Authors note: A.I.D.S. has struck 1,601 people as of June 1983 and it has killed 614 of them.

[8]Henig, *New York Times Magazine*.

[9]West, *Science 83*.

CHAPTER II
The Medical
Definition of A.I.D.S.

According to Dr. Lawrence Mass, in his article in the *New York Native*:

"There is considerable disagreement about the exact definition of A.I.D.S. For some observers, only patients who have already experienced such serious complications of acquired immune deficiency as KS, PCP, or other major opportunistic infections, qualify for the diagnosis of A.I.D.S. Most, however, believe that persistent laboratory evidence of immune deficiency, accompanied by one or more of the symptoms listed below, may also qualify for the diagnosis of A.I.D.S. What is crucial to emphasize here is that many of those with immune deficiency do not yet have and may never develop KS, PCP or other life-threatening complications of A.I.D.S."[1]

The Medical Definition of A.I.D.S. used by the Centers for Disease Control, U. S. Department of Health and Human Services, Public Health Service, Atlanta, Georgia, is as follows:

"The Centers for Disease Control defines a case of acquired immune deficiency syndrome (A.I.D.S.) as a person who has had a reliably diagnosed disease that is strongly suggestive of an underlying cellular immune deficiency but who, at the same time, has had no known underlying cause of cellular immune deficiency nor any other cause of reduced resistance reported to be associated with that disease.

This general case definition may be made more explicit by specifying the particular diseases considered strongly suggestive of cellular immune deficiency and the known causes of cellular immune deficiency or other causes of reduced resistance reported to be associated with particular dieseases. This is done below:

I. **Diseases strongly suggestive of underlying Cellular Immune Deficiency:** These are listed below in 5 etiological categories:
    (A) protozoal and helminthic,
    (B) fungal,
    (C) bacterial,
    (D) viral, and
    (E) cancer.

Within each category, the diseases are listed in alphabetical order. 'Disseminated infection' refers to involvement of liver, bone marrow, or multiple organs, not simply involvement of lungs and multiple lymph nodes. The required diagnostic methods with positive results are shown in parentheses.

A. *Protozoal and Helminthic infections:*
1. Cryptosporidiosis, intestinal, causing diarrhea for over 1 month (on histology or stool microscopy);
2. Pneumocystis carinii pneumonia (on histology, or microscopy of a 'touch' preparation or bronchial washings);
3. Strongyloidosis, causing pneumonia, central nervous system infection, or disseminated infection (on histology);
4. Toxoplasmosis, causing pneumonia or central nervous system infection (on histology or microscopy of a 'touch' preparation).

B. *Fungal Infections:*
1. Aspergillosis, causing central nervous system or disseminated infection (on culture or histology);
2. Candidiasis, causing esophagitis (on histology or microscopy of a 'wet' preparation from the esophagus or endoscopic findings of white plaques on an erythematous mucosal base);
3. Coccidioidomycosis, causing disseminated or central nervous system infection (on culture or histology);
4. Cryptococcosis, causing pulmonary, central nervous system, or disseminated infection (on culture, antigen detection, histology or India ink preparation of CSF);
5. Histoplasmosis, causing disseminated or central nervous system infection (on culture or histology).

C. *Bacterial Infections:*
1. 'Atypical' mycobacteriosis (species other than tuberculosis or lepra), causing disseminated infection (on culture);
2. Nocardiosis (on culture or histology).

D. *Viral Infections:*
1. Cytomegalovirus, causing pulmonary, gastrointestinal tract, or central nervous system infection (on histology);
2. Herpes simplex virus, causing chronic mucocutaneous infection with ulcers persisting more than one month, or pulmonary, gastrointestinal tract, or disseminated infection (on culture, histology or cytology);
3. Progressive multifocal leukoencephalopathy (presumed to be caused by Papovavirus) (on histology).

E. *Cancer:*
1. Kaposi's sarcoma (on histology);
2. Lymphoma limited to the brain (on histology).

II. **Known Causes of Reduced Resistance:** Known causes of reduced resistance to diseases suggestive of immune deficiency are listed in the left column while the diseases that may be attributable to these causes (rather than to the immune deficiency of A.I.D.S.) are listed on the right:

Known Causes of Reduced Resistance	Diseases Possibly Attributable to the Known Causes of Reduced Resistance
1. Systemic corticosteriod or other immuno-suppressive or cytotoxic therapy	Any infection that began during or within one month after such therapy, if the therapy began before signs or symptoms specific for the infected anatomic sites (e.g., dyspnea for pneumonia, headache for encephalitis, diarrhea for colitis); or cancer diagnosed during or within one month after *more than four months* of such therapy, if the therapy began before signs or symptoms specific for the anatomic sites of the cancer.
2. Widely spread cancer of lymphoid or histiocytic tissue, such as lymphoma, Hodgkin's disease, lymphocytic leukemia, or multiple myeloma; (this does not include cancer that is entirely localized to one site, such as primary lymphoma of the brain)	Any other cancer or infection, regardless of whether diagnosed before or after (because a lymphoma may have been present before, even if diagnosed after).
3. Age 60 years or older at diagnosis	Kaposi's sarcoma
4. Age under 28 days (neonatal) at diagnosis	Toxoplasmosis, cytomegalovirus, or herpes simplex virus infections
5. An immune deficiency atypical of A.I.D.S., such as one involving hypogammaglobulinemia; or an immune deficiency of which the cause appears to be a genetic or developmental defect (e.g., thymic dysplasia)[2]	Any infection or cancer diagnosed during such immune deficiency

CHAPTER II FOOTNOTES

[1]Mass, "Basic Questions," *New York Native.*

[2]The U. S. Department of Health and Human Services, Public Health Service/Centers for Disease Control, "*The Case Definition of A.I.D.S. Used by CDC for Epidemiologic Surveillance,*" Atlanta, p. 1, 2, 3.

CHAPTER III
Symptoms of A.I.D.S.

"The first signs of A.I.D.S. can be so innocuous they might be overlooked.[1] "Certain physical signs are suggestive of an underlying immunological disorder. Some of the A.I.D.S. symptoms are subtle and can be mistaken for simple, everyday ailments:

- Low grade, persistent fever, night sweats, dry coughs that are not related to a cold or to smoking

- Shortness of breath with minor exertion

- Loss of weight that is not related to dieting or increase in physical activity

- Extreme fatigue

- Blurred vision, persistent and severe headaches

- Swollen lymph nodes in the neck or under the arms that are not linked to a transient infection of known origin

- Creamy-white patches on the tongue

- Persistent or recurrent itching around the anus

- Diarrhea, bloody stools or gastrointestinal upset that does not go away

- Cuts and infections that do not heal as quickly as usual

- Skin rashes or discolorations that don't go away and may get larger

- And, the symptoms of Kaposi's sarcoma: recently appearing, purple, blue or pink spots or hard nodules on top or beneath the skin that do not disappear, may get larger, and cannot be written off as bruises, blood blisters, insect bites or pimples."[2]

9

"Sometimes the patient is troubled by a common infection that he cannot shake — most typically, shingles or oral thrush (a fungal infection of the mouth and throat). Abdominal cramps may also occur.

Because A.I.D.S. can begin so benignly, homosexual men in apparent good health are flocking to clinics and doctors' offices to see whether they have a hidden case of A.I.D.S."[3]

CHAPTER III FOOTNOTES

[1]Henig, *New York Times Magazine.*

[2]Kaposi's Sarcoma Foundation, "Kaposi's Sarcoma."

[3]Henig, *New York Times Magazine.*

CHAPTER IV
Who Gets A.I.D.S.?

A.I.D.S. does not appear to be a risk to the general public, but because its cause is unknown, this is not yet certain.[1]

"Who gets A.I.D.S.? Victims have belonged primarily to the following four groups: homosexuals, drug addicts, Haitians and hemophiliacs."[2]

"While A.I.D.S. has continued to rage in big-city homosexual communities with terrifying and deadly results, it has also struck Haitian men and women, intravenous-drug users, female partners of drug users, infants and children. It has also struck at least 70 people in no known risk group. A.I.D.S. has become the second leading cause of death — after uncontrollable bleeding in hemophiliacs, and, most recently, a number of surgical patients who have received blood transfusions have contracted A.I.D.S., raising fears among some observers about the nation's blood supply.

As the syndrome spread from the homosexual community to other groups, however, early theories that attempted to explain the outbreak among homosexuals were discarded. Within months, intravenous drug users — both men and women — who were not homosexuals were showing the same signs of immune suppression and developing the same unusual opportunistic infections. Then came Haitians, in both the United States and Haiti, who said they were neither homosexuals nor drug users but who developed what appeared to be an identical syndrome of acquired immune deficiency.

The Haitian connection was made almost by a fluke. An epidemiologist working for the Centers for Disease Control on another matter had trained in Haiti and returned there on vacation. He mentioned to a former colleague the odd infections that were turning up among Haitians in Miami. To his astonishment, the Haitian dermatologist replied that he, too, had seen several cases of Kaposi's sarcoma. Since then, teams of physicians from the Centers for Disease Control and from the University of Miami, where many Haitian immigrants with A.I.D.S. are treated, have visited Haiti in an attempt to confirm that it really is the same syndrome and to determine if the agent originated in the Caribbean and moved north or whether it was transported to Haiti from this country.

Haitian A.I.D.S. victims are often involved in voodoo and spiritualism, but it isn't known what in their rituals might be relevant to the transmission of A.I.D.S."[3]

"Very little is known about risk factors for Haitians with A.I.D.S."[4]

"In the spring of 1982, the Centers for Disease Control received its first reports of A.I.D.S. in hemophiliacs. Some of these patients were probably exposed to the A.I.D.S. agent in a blood-clotting medication called Factor VIII concentrate that is made from the blood of thousands of donors. Anywhere from 2,500 to 22,000 blood donors are used to make just one lot of this widely used product; one lot treats

11

about 100 patients. To date, the Centers for Disease Control has received a total of eight confirmed reports of hemophiliacs with A.I.D.S., six of whom have died. All used Factor VIII concentrate rather than an older, less convenient blood product called cryoprecipitate, which is made from the blood of a handful of donors. In view of the A.I.D.S. threat, some hemophilia experts are urging a return to cryoprecipitate, especially in mild or newly diagnosed cases.

In the summer of 1982, the Centers for Disease Control received reports of three patients who contracted A.I.D.S. after receiving blood transfusions. Two of those patients were adults from the Northeast and the third was an infant in San Francisco who needed a transfusion to correct an Rh-factor incompatibility. Four more cases of possible transmission of A.I.D.S. through blood transfusions are now being investigated.

By mid-January, the Centers for Disease Control had received five reports of A.I.D.S. that had spread to female sexual partners of drug abusers. In four of those cases, the male partners had not even been sick. Thus, A.I.D.S. qualified as a sexually transmitted disease among heterosexuals. It also began to be clear that individuals could be identified who might be carriers of the A.I.D.S. agent, able to infect other people without themselves developing symptoms."[5]

Susan West, in her article in *Science 83*, reported:

"Right now, the attention is on two new groups of victims. The first is women who are sexual partners of men with A.I.D.S., adding support to the belief that A.I.D.S. is passed by sexual contact. The second group is children.

As of mid-January, 26 children less than five years old appear to have come down with the syndrome; 10 have died. None have Kaposi's but they have pneumocystis and other infections and the characteristic immune system breakdown. Most of the children have parents who are Haitian, drug users, or who have had homosexual contact. Some of the parents have A.I.D.S.; others could be carriers. No one knows if the children pick it up in their mothers' wombs or from the intimate relationship of parent and infant. But more than ever, A.I.D.S. appears to be infectious."[6]

"The groups most recently found to be at risk for A.I.D.S. present a particularly poignant problem. Innocent bystanders caught in the path of a new disease, that can make no behavioral decisions to minimize their risk: hemophiliacs cannot stop taking blood-clotting medication; surgery patients cannot stop getting transfusions; women cannot control the drug habits of their mates; babies cannot choose their mothers."[7]

According to the U. S. Department of Health and Human Services in their Morbidity and Mortality Weekly Report dated March 4, 1982, no A.I.D.S. cases have been documented among health care or laboratory personnel caring for A.I.D.S. patients or processing laboratory specimens. To date, no person-to-person transmission has been identified other than through intimate contact or blood transfusion.

CHAPTER IV FOOTNOTES

[1] U. S. Department of Health and Human Services, "Questions and Answers."

[2] Lawrence Mass, M.D., "Gays and Bad Blood: No Scapegoating — Yet," *New York Native*, III, no. 4, (17 - 30 January 1982), p. 25.

[3] Henig, *New York Times Magazine*, pp. 30, 31.

[4] Centers for Disease Control, "Prevention of Acquired Immune Deficiency Syndrome (A.I.D.S.): Report of Inter-Agency Recommendations," *Morbidity and Mortality Weekly Report*, XXXII, no. 8, (4 March 1983), p. 101.

[5] Henig, *New York Times Magazine*, p. 31.

[6] Susan West, "One Step Behind A Killer," *Science 83*, IV, No. 2 (March 1983), p. 44.

[7] Henig, *New York Times Magazine*, p. 36.

CHAPTER V
History of the
Current Outbreak
of A.I.D.S.

"Medical investigators have traced in broad outline the spread of A.I.D.S.

In the spring of 1981, clinicians in New York City began to see a surprising number of cases of Kaposi's sarcoma.

Kaposi' sarcoma in its classic form, as it is usually seen in this country, is treatable; its victims usually live at least 10 years after the condition is diagnosed and they often die of other causes. So, when clinics in New York began to report severe cases of the rare sarcoma in young men, the medical community was alarmed.

At about the same time, infectious-disease specialists throughout New York were noticing another bizarre occurrence. At the weekly city-wide infectious-disease meetings sponsored by the New York City Department of Health, where physicians present their most perplexing cases, many of the cases mentioned involved the severe and potentially lethal form of pneumonia, Pneumocystic carinii.

Like Kaposi's sarcoma, Pneumocystic pneumonia also affected patients whose immune systems were severely compromised: cancer-chemotherapy patients and organ transplant recipients.

Now, a new group of patients was developing the disease. Eleven cases of Pneumocystis in young men were found. Within a year of diagnosis, eight of the 11 men were dead.

In mid-1981, the Federal Government became involved in the mystery. To investigate the outbreak, the CDC formed a special task force which published its first findings in June and July in Morbidity and Mortality Weekly Report (see Appendix C), CDC's official publication. Of the 116 homosexual patients identified at the time, about 30 percent had Kaposi's sarcoma, about 50 percent had Pneumocystis pneumonia and about 10 percent had both. The remaining 10 percent had unusual infections that also usually affect only the immunosuppressed.

Half of the victims lived in New York City and there was a large concentration of cases in California. Those studied were sexually promiscuous: they frequented homosexual bars and bathhouses (where a typical visit may include sex with 15 to 20 deliberately anonymous men). Many of them also used 'poppers,' inhalant amyl nitrite and butyl nitrite.

In the fall of 1981, the CDC studied the sexual habits of 50 homosexual victims of A.I.D.S.

For 13 A.I.D.S. victims in Los Angeles, a list was compiled of all the sex partners that the A.I.D.S. victims or their survivors could name for the previous five years. They then compared those names with the roster of all the cases in the country. The result: Of those 13 cases, nine had sex contacts in common, a finding that could not possibly have been a random coincidence. This was the so-called L.A. cluster of A.I.D.S. patients. Later, a missing link was found between Los Angeles and New York. An A.I.D.S. victim from New York was identified as having been a sexual partner of four men in the L.A. cluster — as well as of four other men in New York who also developed A.I.D.S."[1]

"One cannot presume that this is the first epidemic of A.I.D.S. in history. Since the ability of medical science to detect indicators of immunosuppression is relatively recent, one must ask:

(1) How long have there been individuals with collapsed immune systems; and

(2) How long have such individuals been recognized and observed in classic epidemiologic terms?

It is possible that immunosuppression has existed for as long as there have been viruses; admittedly, there is no way to verify this hypothesis. However, review of autopsy reports in the United States going back thirty years has indicated the possibility that A.I.D.S. may have existed in a limited fashion as early as 1950.

Verification of these reports as evidence of A.I.D.S. is impossible since the tests which detect immune deficiency have only recently come into use. However, the cases referred to in the autopsy reports bear such striking resemblance to A.I.D.S., which most are claiming is a new phenomenon, that it now seems quite likely that A.I.D.S. has occurred in the United States and other countries before, but has only recently been recognized.

The heroic hunt for mutant viruses has been a response in previous epidemics when the ministrations of doctors remained ineffective. In the winter of 1978-79, an outbreak of fatal respiratory infections among children in Naples, Italy was initially believed to have been caused by some new, mutant virus. Eventually, the mystery was solved: 'Naples disease' proved to be the result of immunological abnormalities caused by 'socioeconomic factors, such as malnutrition and family size, and a transitory immunosuppression due to vaccination.'

Presumably, the present epidemic of A.I.D.S. among promiscuous urban gay males is occurring because of the unprecedented promiscuity of the last ten to fifteen years. The commercialization of promiscuity and the explosion of establishments such as bathhouses, bookstores and backrooms is unique in western history. It has been mass participation in this lifestyle that has led to the creation of an increasingly disease-polluted pool of sexual partners — which many feel has in turn very likely led to the present epidemic of A.I.D.S."[2]

CHAPTER V FOOTNOTES

[1]Henig, *New York Times Magazine*, pp. 30, 31.

[2]Michael Callen, Richard Berkowitz, Richard Dworkin, "We Know Who We Are — Two Gay Men Declare War on Promiscuity," *New York Native*, II, no. 25 (8 - 21 November 1982), p. 25.

CHAPTER VI
What Causes A.I.D.S.?

Investigators have not yet been able to find the cause, or causes, of the loss of immunity found in A.I.D.S. victims. The occurrence of the syndrome among hemophilia patients suggests the possibility of transmission of an agent through blood products, but this has not been proved. One leading hypothesis is that the causative agent is a blood-borne virus. Risk factors that have been suggested from studies to date include an increased number of sexual partners for homosexual men and sharing of needles for those using illicit drugs, but as yet there is no definitive explanation.[1]

"The continuing search for a cause is leading scientists in several directions at once. Researchers are particularly interested in two viruses, both of them herpes virus: cytomegalovirus (CMV) and Epstein-Barr virus. CMV, which causes mental and motor retardation in children infected before birth, has been know to suppress the immune system in mice. In addition, CMV antibodies were found in 80 to 95 percent of A.I.D.S. patients, compared with 50 percent in the general population. Antibodies for Epstein-Barr virus, which causes infectious mononucleosis, were also found in extremely high concentrations in A.I.D.S. patients. Patients with A.I.D.S. sometimes show Epstein-Barr antibody levels '10-fold to 100-fold higher than normal.'

As early as 1979, 5 to 10 hemophiliacs a year were dying of unusual infections and cancers that today would be called A.I.D.S., although the disease had not yet been identified. Anti-clotting medication itself might have an imune-suppressant effect."[2]

"There is a theory that sperm can be immunosuppressive and a possible contributing factor in some cases of A.I.D.S.[3] The current etiological candidate for A.I.D.S. is a new infectious agent. However, many feel that it is unlikely that this complex syndrome is the result of a single factor and investigators should consider additional possibilities.

There are at least two ways in which allogenetic leukocytes (T-lymphocytes and other white blood cells from a sexual partner) could cause immune suppression. In the first, foreign leukocytes that are themselves immunosuppressive may reach the bloodstream of passive partners by way of the kinds of tiny cuts and abrasions that are believed to occur frequently during anal intercourse. In the second, some of these foreign leukocytes may contain active viruses such as CMV and may be initiating repetitive cycles of viral-induced immune suppression.

There is one gaping flaw in the sperm theory. It cannot explain the appearance of A.I.D.S. in the non-gay groups, nor does it explain why this disease has not been seen in this population or in female prostitutes before. Although it is likely that all populations of patients with A.I.D.S. have been exposed to at least one etiologic common denominator, it is also likely that not all etiologic factors are identical, since Kaposi's sarcoma appears to be limited to the homosexual population. Thus, allogenetic leukocytes as well as a virus could be a factor in the development of A.I.D.S. among homosexuals."[4]

To date, the exact cause of A.I.D.S. must be recorded as. . . .

"unknown."

CHAPTER VI FOOTNOTES

[1]U. S. Department of Health and Human Services, "Questions and Answers."

[2]Henig, *New York Times Magazine*, pp. 31, 36, 42.

[3]In animals, sperm in the bloodstream is known to suppress the immune system.

[4]Larry Kramer, "1,112 and Counting," *New York Native*, III, no. 8, (14 - 27 March 1983), p. 17, col. 4.

CHAPTER VII
Promiscuity, Gays and A.I.D.S.

"There is overwhelming evidence that the present health crisis of A.I.D.S. is a direct result of excessive promiscuity.

What is meant by 'excessive promiscuity?' The National Cancer Institute, using figures provided by the Centers for Disease Control, stated in March 1982:

> *The median number of lifetime male sexual partners for homosexual male patients (with A.I.D.S.) is 1,160.*

Few have been willing to say it so clearly but the single greatest risk factor for contacting A.I.D.S. seems to be a history of multiple male homosexual sexual contacts with partners who are having multiple male homosexual sexual contacts.

What has been missing so far in the investigation of the health crisis has been the informed opinions of those who have created it. Can researchers really comprehend the dynamics of urban gay male promiscuity? Can they understand the health implications for a 27-year-old who has had 2,000 sexual partners? Or 1,000? Or even 500?

These are the gay men who are becoming the victims of A.I.D.S.

Some have concluded that there is no mutant virus and there will be no vaccine. Promiscuous gays must accept the fact that they have overloaded their immune systems with common viruses and other sexually transmitted infections. Their lifestyle has created the present epidemic of A.I.D.S. among gay men. But, in the end, whichever theory you choose to believe, the obvious and immediate solution to the present crisis is the end of urban homosexual male promiscuity as it is known today.

Following are some statements taken from personal experiences of A.I.D.S. victims, from consultations with various researchers and physicians, from support groups for A.I.D.S. victims, from health crisis groups in New York City and San Francisco, and from both the medical and the lay press.

Some believe that it is the *accumulation of risk* through leading a promiscuous gay urban lifestyle which has led to the breakdown of immune responses that we are seeing now. Most published medical reports indicate that continued re-exposure and reinfection with common viruses (most notably cytomegalovirus), in conjunction with other common venereal infections and perhaps other factors, had led to the present health crisis among urban gay promiscuous men.

Every sexually active gay man knows that he is much more likely to pick up any of a variety of sexually transmitted diseases today than he was five years ago. Five years ago, who'd ever heard of amebas? Herpes now makes the cover of popular magazines. In retrospect, these epidemics were signaling the coming of a major health crisis.

The gay men who are developing A.I.D.S. have long histories of many sexually transmitted diseases. These include amebiasis; hepatitis A, B, and non-A, non-B; venereal warts; penile, anal, and oral gonorrhea; syphilis; herpes simplex types 1 and 2 non-specific urethritis and proctitis. It appears that venereal disease has been defined too narrowly. Many viruses can and have been transmitted during sex and we must now add cytomegalovirus (CMV) and Epstein-Barr, among others, to the list of sexually transmitted diseases which urban gay males have been trading at an unprecedented rate over the last decade.

In one study published in the *New England Journal of Medicine*, 94 percent of sexually active gay men tested showed evidence of CMV infection and 14 percent were actively contagious for CMV at the time of testing. Some believe that the prevalence of CMV is the major link in the process of developing A.I.D.S. among gay men.

Many CMV infections are asymptomatic, which means that an individual may have CMV and be immunosuppressed without even knowing it. There is a high risk for picking up the many bacterial, fungal, amebic and particularly viral infections in promiscuity.

One can be reinfected with CMV. No one knows for certain what the immunological results of re-infection are but since a single infection with CMV can be immunosuppressive, it is easy to imagine what the cumulative effects of re-exposure to CMV and other infections might be.

Simply stated, gays that live in or frequent New York, San Francisco, Los Angeles, or any of several other metropolitan areas, will more than likely be having sex with men who are sick. Those that have sex with sick men may get sick too — not with any new diseases but again and again with CMV and other common infections. Sooner or later, they simply will not recover.

Other factors may contribute to the development of A.I.D.S. in promiscuous gay men, including stress, diet, intravenous or other drug usage, the possible immunosuppressive consequences of sperm and seminal fluid, and excessive exposure to ultraviolet light. However, none of these contributing factors would be sufficient alone to cause A.I.D.S.; it is the widespread, repeated re-exposure and reinfection with common viruses that has set the stage for the epidemic of A.I.D.S. that we are now witnessing."[1]

CHAPTER VII FOOTNOTE

[1]Callen, *New York Native.*

CHAPTER VIII
Where Is the Outbreak?

Between June 1981 and June 1983, over 1,600 cases of acquired immune deficiency syndrome have been reported to the Centers for Disease Control from 34 states, the District of Columbia and 15 countries.[1]

The geographical distribution of reported cases of A.I.D.S. has been unusual, with over half the reported cases from New York City and about 22 percent from California.[2]

See chart below.[3]

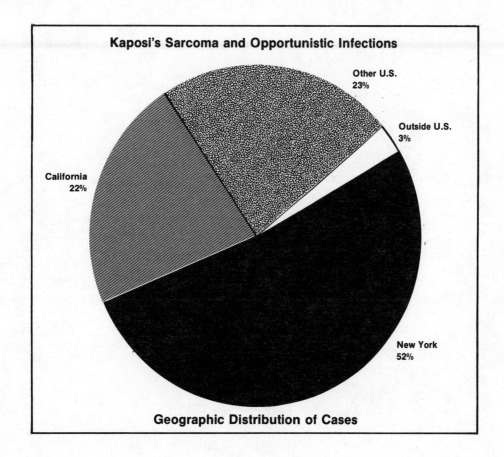

Kaposi's Sarcoma and Opportunistic Infections

Other U.S. 23%

Outside U.S. 3%

California 22%

New York 52%

Geographic Distribution of Cases

CHAPTER VIII FOOTNOTES

[1]Centers for Disease Control, *Morbidity and MOrtality Weekly Report*, "Prevention of AIDS."

[2]U. S. Department of Health and Human Services, "Questions and Answers."

[3]Lawrence Mass, M.D., "Congress Looks at the Epidemic," *New York Native*, II, no. 12 (10 - 23 May 1982), p. 17.

CHAPTER IX
Mortality Rate Of A.I.D.S. Victims

"A.I.D.S. has a very high fatality rate, ranging from 20 percent to as high as 70 percent depending upon the opportunistic disease. Centers for Disease Control investigators do not know of any patient with A.I.D.S. who has regained lost immunity.

A.I.D.S. is deadly."[1] According to Dr. James Allen of the A.I.D.S. Activity Department, Centers for Disease Control in Atlanta, Georgia, as of June 14, 1983 there have been 1,601 cases of A.I.D.S. reported. Of those, 614 have died. Of the cases reported before June 1981, 75 percent are dead. Although these earlier cases probably received less experienced treatment than A.I.D.S. patients get today, some fear that the five-year death rate will be higher than 86 percent. Smallpox, by comparison, killed 25 percent of its victims.[2]

"It has been reported that one in every 360 gay men in San Francisco has A.I.D.S. Of the 200 cases diagnosed in San Francisco, 53 have died."[3]

CHAPTER IX FOOTNOTES

[1] Henig, *New York Times Magazine*.

[2] U. S. Department of Health and Human Services, "Questions and Answers."

[3] Marty Gonzales, "A.I.D.S.," TV News Documentary, KCRA-TV, Channel 3(Sacramento), 11:00 p.m. News, March 23, 1983.

CHAPTER X
A.I.D.S. and Guilt

"The grisly toll is mounting: over 1,600 cases of A.I.D.S. world-wide, almost half of them in the New York area, hundreds of them fatal, many, perhaps all, of the rest expected to be so. Young men are dying of this terminal illness all over.

What makes this death uniquely difficult to accept? Aunt Tillie did no more to bring on her breast cancer than to be a woman. She is seen as a victim, pure and simple. Though her tumor involves an organ intimately connected with sex, there is no shame associated with it. Breast cancer is a source of endless discussion in the press.

Leukemia victims are the darlings of the world of terminal illness. There's nothing like leukemia to arouse sympathy and support and compassion — Love Story and Ronald McDonald House, etc. The innocent leukemia patient at times seems to have a certain pride in his or her affliction.

With A.I.D.S., there's guilt. You don't have to know a thing about the postulated cause of it to feel the guilt in the air: the hospital doors with isolation signs posted all over them; the gowns, the gloves, the masks; the rapidity with which the nurses shut the door when they must go in or out. Everyone knows by now that promiscuity and A.I.D.S. are somehow all tied in together, aren't they? We've all heard the stories of the incredible numbers of sexual contacts, the quantities of drugs consumed, the venerally transmitted diseases sustained by the average victim of A.I.D.S. and in the United States, the only thing worse than promiscuity is gay promiscuity. The idea that A.I.D.S. is the wrath of God come down on homosexuals for their evil ways is widespread. Gay men have always believed that they have something to be ashamed of. This is instilled in every homosexual.

But what happens to the ego of the victim of A.I.D.S. lying in his hospital bed? Patients regress when they are sick. He's in an isolated room in a hospital, lacking privacy nonetheless, with all of his bodily functions gone haywire and being closely monitored by strangers. Just a few short months ago, he was perfectly healthy.

What do the healthy ones do with this guilt? Weird things; different things. Some become obsessed with the idea that they have A.I.D.S. themselves, all evidence to the contrary. They make repeated visits to their doctor, to other doctors and to therapists, if they get onto the right track. These people are miserable and their guilt is a purely personal burden."[1]

"Suicides are now being reported of men who would rather die than face medical uncertainty, uncertain therapies, hospital treatment and the appalling statistic that 86 percent of all serious A.I.D.S. victims die after three years' time."[2]

Hand-in-hand with all of the terrible physical symptoms the A.I.D.S. victim has to endure, is the definite presence of guilt and the additional problems that guilt adds to their illness.

CHAPTER X FOOTNOTES

[1]Peter A. Seitzman, M.D., "Guilt and A.I.D.S.," *New York Native*, III, no. 3, (3 - 16 January 1983), p. 23.

[2]Kramer, *New York Native*, p. 1.

CHAPTER XI
What is Being Done to Combat A.I.D.S.?

The Centers for Disease Control formed a task force in July 1981 to investigate the problem of A.I.D.S. and seek methods of control and prevention. Workers on the task force include physicians, public health advisors, epidemiologists, statisticians, laboratory scientists and others both at the Centers for Disease Control headquarters in Atlanta and stationed at Centers for Disease Control facilities and State and local health departments across the country. As a public health agency, Centers for Disease Control goals are to discover the causative agent of A.I.D.S. and to interrupt its transmission. Centers for Disease Control also assists clinical centers in developing and evaluating treatments for A.I.D.S. patients.[1]

Activities of Centers for Disease Control include surveillance, epidemiologic studies and laboratory investigations. A surveillance system has been implemented to receive and solicit case reports from physicians and health departments, and surveillance of hemophilia treatment centers is being planned. Among the epidemiologic investigations in homosexual populations have been a case-control study in New York and California and an analysis of clusters of sexually related cases. These studies support the hypothesis of sexual transmission of an infectious agent. Studies are also being done of homosexual cases outside New York and California, apparently healthy homosexual men with "subclinical immunosuppression," heterosexual cases and chronic lymphadenopathy patients to identify other potential risk factors for KS and opportunistic infections. Investigations and studies of cases among Haitians are being conducted in Haiti and the United States.

Intensive laboratory studies include injections of tissue from several sources of patients into multiple cell cultures and laboratory animals, including rodents and non-human primates; observation of these cultures and animals; and prolonged immunologic and pathologic follow-up of the laboratory animals. Extensive laboratory investigations of patient materials (lymphocytes, lymph nodes, autopsy specimens) are being conducted through the use of highly technical methods, including electron microscopy and various immunofluorescent techniques. Examination of blood products such as Factor VIII concentrate and cryoprecipitate, used by hemophiliacs, is underway.

Information gathered about the epidemic has been shared with the medical and public health community through presentations at public and scientific meetings and the publication of ten Morbidity and Mortality Weekly Report articles (see Appendix C).

Centers for Disease Control activities are being coordinated with other Public Health Services agencies, including the National Institutes of Health and the Food and Drug Administration, as well as State and local health departments, and academicians and clinicians providing care for these patients.[2]

Elsewhere that are many groups working to solve this problem, including international, federal, state and local public health agencies, private and public foundations, numerous medical schools and research institutes, individual health practitioners and others both here and in other countries.[3]

"As A.I.D.S. threatens to move into mainstream America, efforts to find its cause and stop its spread have intensified. In January, Congress allocated $2 million to the Centers for Disease Control for A.I.D.S. research. Homosexual communities in major cities have set up support groups that provide information and guidance for victims and raise money for research. Hemophiliacs, many of whom depend on a clotting agent gathered from the blood of thousands of donors, have recently recommended that those at risk for A.I.D.S. be eliminated from the donor pool. Though the moral and legal implications of such screening have yet to be determined, blood suppliers are re-examining their procedures and the Department of Health and Human Services is working on proposals that would provide stricter screening of blood donors.

The search for the A.I.D.S. agent is being coordinated in Atlanta, at the Centers for Disease Control. There, 20 full-time physicians and other professionals (with help from 80 professionals working part-time) canvass the four corners of the outbreak — New York, San Francisco, Los Angeles and Miami. They also keep track of the laboratory and clinical experiments being mounted not only at the Centers for Disease Control but also at research hospitals across the country. The job of these medical sleuths is complicated by the unusual nature of the patients.

Investigators are following groups of apparently healthy patients with certain immunological abnormalities to see who among them develop opportunistic infections or other more obvious symptoms of A.I.D.S."[4]

"There are 70 cases who don't fit known risk groups and eight of those received blood within several years of the onset of their A.I.D.S. illness. It is this latter unclassified group that has stirred controversy about how to deal with the possibility that A.I.D.S. can be contracted by receiving a blood transfusion taken from an already infected although as yet undiagnosed donor.

The National Hemophilia Foundation has sought a ban on gay male blood donors until the A.I.D.S. mystery is solved and the disease controlled. But the idea has bogged down in practical and constitutional questions. How do you determine who is gay except by asking him and what's to assure that they are telling the truth?"[5]

"There are a number of reasons why the voluntary abstention approach will not work. Because much of this country's donated blood is actually paid for, many 'donors' who need the money, such as drug addicts, will falsely identify themselves when screened. In the case of gay people, the escalation of homophobia in this country is more likely to have a paradoxical effect on this situation. That is, some gay men, fearful of losing their jobs or other persecutions, may feel pressured to donate blood during community or office blood drives as a way of proving to suspicious colleagues that they are not gay. The Work Group for A.I.D.S. Prevention has adopted a resolution advising health care providers that it is inappropriate to screen potential donors of blood or blood products on the basis of sexual preference."[6]

"At the moment, the three groups most heavily involved in blood programs, the American Association of Blood Banks, the American Red Cross and the Council of Community Blood Centers have arrived at an uneasy compromise policy: donors 'should not be recruited from' the three identified high-risk groups, gay men, Haitians and IV drug abusers. In addition, the questionnaire filled out by donors asks questions relating to A.I.D.S. symptoms."[7]

"Laboratories have stepped up their search for a virus-like organism. The researchers put samples of urine, blood, sputum, and semen from A.I.D.S. patients in cultures designed to coax even the most stubborn virus to grow. They checked each culture under the electron microscope for signs of foreign organisms. They marked antibodies to known viruses with fluorescent dyes and set them loose to see if they would latch onto a new but related virus. They isolated well-known viruses and examined them to see if there was anything new and different about them. They fed the cultures growth factors and concentrated them to make it easier to spot a virus. They injected marmoset monkeys and chimpanzees and mice with samples from the patients to see if the animals would get A.I.D.S. After nearly two years, they've found nothing.

There may be a good reason they haven't. It may be that the virus or organism is long gone by the time a doctor realizes a patient has A.I.D.S. and the laboratory gets specimens. If scientists could find people soon enough, the culprit might still be there. And this presents a vicious circle. It would be nice if there was a test to identify the early stage of the disease, but a test can't be developed until the agent is found. And to isolate an agent, patients must be caught early enough. Patients with the vague syndrome called lymphadenopathy may represent the beginning of the disease and workers are keeping track of some of them to see if they develop full-blown A.I.D.S. But even that stage may not be early enough.

Eventually, someone will study a particularly susceptible population — get them while they are still healthy, follow them and routinely take specimens, watch to see who develops the disease, then go back and look at all their specimens. But it will take hundreds of people to get one case. . . .and, lots of money.

If the epidemiologists can find such a population, if the laboratory researchers can isolate an organism, then maybe they can develop a test to determine who has A.I.D.S. and a vaccine to give those who do — if it's an organism for which a vaccine can be made."[8]

"The University of California at Davis Primate Center is studying Simian A.I.D.S. in monkeys. It has been found that the A.I.D.S. found in the monkeys is the same as the A.I.D.S. found in humans. The monkeys share close intimate contact. The researchers at Davis are working on a breakthrough in the A.I.D.S. disease and they are relying on this link between the A.I.D.S. in humans and A.I.D.S. in monkeys to shed some light on this mysterious disease."[9]

"The Centers for Disease Control is charged by our government to fully monitor all epidemics and unusual diseases.

To learn something from an epidemic you have to keep records and statistics. Statistics come from interviewing victims and getting as much information from them as you can — before they die. To get the best information, you have to ask the right questions.

There have been so many A.I.D.S. victims that the Centers for Disease Control is no longer able to get to them fast enough. It has given up. The National Institutes of Health is also still fielding a questionnaire.

Important, vital case histories are now being lost because of this cessation of Centers for Disease Control interviewing. This is a waste with as terrifying implications as the alarming rise in case numbers and doctors finally admitting they don't know what's going on. As each man dies, as one or both sets of men who had interacted with each other come down with A.I.D.S., yet more information that might reveal patterns of transmissibility is not being monitored and collected and studied. We are being denied perhaps the easiest and fastest research tool available at this moment.

It will require at least $200,000 to prepare a new questionnaire to study the next important question that must be answered: How is A.I.D.S. being transmitted? (In which bodily fluids, by which sexual behaviors, in what social environments?)

For months the Centers for Disease Control has been asked to begin such preparations for continued surveillance. They are so stretched to their limits and dreadfully underfunded for what they are being asked, in all areas, to do."[10]

"The American Association of Physicians for Human Rights has decided to place increased emphasis on the psycho-social impact of acquired immune deficiency syndrome on its victims; the group has also pledged to carry out a more effective policy of educating gay and straight physicians nationally about A.I.D.S.

The actions — which took place at an American Association of Physicians for Human Rights conference held in Boston in mid-October — came in response to recent criticism that the gay medical community is not doing enough to disseminate information and provide psychological support to A.I.D.S. patients.

Sixty gay physicians attended the conference. But there are an estimated 50,000 gay physicians in the United States and American Associations of Physicians for Human Rights members made plans to locate a greater number of these physicians and engage their help in dealing with the epidemic. Members also recognized the need to expand educational programs beyond major metoropolitan areas on the east and west coasts.

Members at the conference agreed on the importance of deemphasizing the rigid medical model in A.I.D.S. treatment (which places importance completely upon treatment of physiological ailments while expanding existing psychosocial support mechanisms. American Association of Physicians for Human Rights plans to set up a national hotline on psychosocial issues, possibly in conjunction with the National Gay Task Force's new national hotline.

The association also made plans to push for further research into A.I.D.S. by the National Institutes of Health and the Centers for Disease Control, to help the Gay Rights National Lobby in its lobbying efforts for funding on Capitol Hill and to urge non-gay medical colleagues to be more active in helping obtain funds for A.I.D.S. research."[11]

CHAPTER XI FOOTNOTES

[1]U. S. Department of Health and Human Services, "Questions and Answers."

[2]U. S. Department of Health and Human Services, Public Health Service/Centers for Disease Control, "Status of Acquired Immune Deficiency Syndrome (A.I.D.S.)," Atlanta, October, 1982.

[3]U. S. Department of Health and Human Services, "Questions and Answers."

[4]Henig, *New York Times Magazine*, pp. 28, 30, 44.

[5]Don Stanley, "A.I.D.S. The Price of Sex?", *The Sacramento Bee*, Scene, 4 January 1983, B5, col. 1-6, B7, col. 1-3.

[6]Mass, "Gays and Bad Blood," *New York Native*, p. 8.

[7]Stanley, *The Sacramento Bee*.

[8]Susan West, *Science 83*, p. 45.

[9]Gonzales, KCRA-TV.

[10]Kramer, *New York Native*, p. 19.

[11]Amarnack, *New York Native*, p. 9.

CHAPTER XII
A.I.D.S. and Politics

"To date, Congress has given a total of $2 million to the Centers for Disease Control in Atlanta to study A.I.D.S. More people have died of this disease in 18 months than the deaths from Legionella and Toxic Shock Syndrome combined. Yet, seven times the amount of money was spent by the government on each of those diseases."[1]

"Following are some remarks by Congressman Henry A. Waxman, Chairman, Subcommittee on Health and the Environment (D-Calif.) at congressional hearings on the recent outbreak of gay-related A.I.D.S.:

'I want to be especially blunt about the political aspects of Kaposi's sarcoma. This horrible disease afflicts members of one of the nation's most stigmatized and discriminated-against minorities. The victims are not typical Main Street Americans. They are gays — mainly from New York, Los Angeles and San Francisco.

There is no doubt in my mind that if the same disease had appeared among Americans of Norwegian descent, or among tennis players, rather than among gay males, the responses of both the government and the medical community would have been different.

Legionnaire's disease hit a group of predominantly white, heterosexual, middle-aged members of the American Legion. The respectability of the victims brought them a degree of attention and funding for research and treatment far greater than that made available so far to the victims of Kaposi's sarcoma. I want to emphasize the contrast because the 'more popular' Legionnaire's disease affected fewer people (and proved less likely to be fatal). What society judged was not the severity of the disease but the social acceptability of the individuals affected with it.

We can't talk about the 'gay cancer.' There is a cancer which seems predominantly to affect gay men, but it is a cancer and a public health concern for all Americans. Above all, I intend to fight any effort by anyone at any level to make public policy regarding Kaposi's sarcoma or any other disease on the basis of his or her personal prejudices regarding other people's sexual preferences or lifestyles.'"[2]

"One cynical explanation of why the A.I.D.S. research doesn't turn up in the federal budget is that avoiding open support for the research keeps the A.I.D.S. problem identified with our present administration, saving them from having to face anti-gay New Right supporters, who targeted the last $2 million appropriation as a bonus won by 'militant homosexuals' who could be disease-free if they changed their sexual lifestyles. Presumably, current budget writers weren't anxious to appear to be the newest captives of the militant homosexual lobby."[3]

"For over a year and a half the National Institutes of Health has been 'reviewing' which from among some $55 million worth of grant applications for A.I.D.S. research money it will eventually fund.

It's not even a question of the National Institutes of Health having to ask Congress for money. It's already there — waiting. The National Institutes of Health has almost $8 million already appropriated that it has yet to release into usefulness.

There is no question that if this epidemic were happening to the straight, white, non-intravenous drug-using, middle-class community, that money would have been put into use almost two years ago when the first alarming signs of this epidemic were noticed.

During the first *two weeks* of the Tylenol scare, the government spent *$10 million* to find out what was happening."[4]

In the June 14, 1983 edition of the Sacramento Union, it was reported by the Associated Press that "a $30 million fund to deal with the A.I.D.S. epidemic and other public health emergencies had been approved in a bill by the House. The measure, passed by voice vote, is opposed by the Reagan administration. The Senate is considering a similar bill."[5] The article states that, "In recent years, unexpected health crises have been of such numbers, size and complexity that contingency funds have been exhausted and the PHS has been forced to pursue alternate courses, said a report by the House Energy and Commerce Committee.

The Public Health Service has diverted funds from other activities, asked for supplemental appropriations or 'been forced by fiscal limitations to respond unevenly or with minimal resources, allowing crises to continue longer and more broadly,' the report continued. The administration argues that the Department of Health and Human Services already has adequate authority to deal with public health emergencies."[6]

CHAPTER XII FOOTNOTES

[1] Don Stanley, "A.I.D.S. Nightmare: Puzzling, Deadly — And Spreading," *The Sacramento Bee*, Scene, 4 January 1983, A18, col. 1-6, A19, col. 3,4.

[2] Ron Vachon, "If KS Had Hit Tennis Players," *New York Native*, II, no. 11, 26 April-9 May 1982, p. 11.

[3] Larry Bush, "Reagan Playing Shell Games with A.I.D.S. Funding," *New York Native*, III, no. 6, (14 - 27 February 1983), pp. 9, 10.

[4] Kramer, *New York Native*, p. 19. (italics author's)

[5]*The Sacramento Union (AP)*, June 14, 1983, p. 1.

[6]Ibid.

CHAPTER XIII
Prevention and Control of A.I.D.S.

Statements on prevention and control of A.I.D.S. have been issued by the National Gay Task Force, the National Hemophilia Foundation, the American Red Cross, the American Association of Blood Banks, the Council of Community Blood Centers, the American Association of Physicians for Human Rights and others. These groups agree that steps should be implemented to reduce the potential risk of transmitting A.I.D.S. through blood products but differ in the methods proposed to accomplish this goal. Public health agencies, community organizations and medical organizations and groups share the responsibility to rapidly disseminate information on A.I.D.S. and recommended precautions.

Although the cause of A.I.D.S. remains unknown, the Public Health Service recommends the following actions:

1. Sexual contact should be avoided with persons known or suspected to have A.I.D.S. Members of high risk groups should be aware that multiple sexual partners increase the probability of developing A.I.D.S.

2. As a temporary measure, members of groups at increased risk for A.I.D.S. should refrain from donating plasma and/or blood. This recommendation includes all individuals belonging to such groups, even though many individuals are at little risk of A.I.D.S. Centers collecting plasma and/or blood should inform potential donors of this recommendation. The Food and Drug Administration (FDA) is preparing new recommendations for manufacturers of plasma derivatives and for establishiments collecting plasma or blood. This is an interim measure to protect recipients of blood products and blood until specific laboratory tests are available.

3. Studies should be conducted to evaluate screening procedures for their effectiveness in identifying and excluding plasma and blood with a high probability of transmitting A.I.D.S. These procedures should include specific laboratory tests as well as careful histories and physical examinations.

4. Physicians should adhere strictly to medical indications for transfusions, and autologous blood transfusions are encouraged.

5. Work should continue toward development of safer blood products for use by hemophilia

patients.

The National Hemophilia Foundation has made specific recommendations for management of patients with hemophilia.

The interim recommendation requesting that high-risk persons refrain from donating plasma and/or blood is especially important for donors whose plasma is recovered from plasmapheresis centers or other sources and pooled to make products that are not inactivated and may transmit infections, such as hepatitis B. The clear intent of this recommendation is to eliminate plasma and blood potentially containing the putative A.I.D.S. agent from the supply. Since no specific test is known to detect A.I.D.S. at an early stage in a potential donor, the recommendation to discourage donation must encompass all members of groups at increased risk for A.I.D.S., even though it includes many individuals who may be at little risk of transmitting A.I. D. S.

As long as the cause remains unknown, the ability to understand the natural history of A.I.D.S. and to undertake preventive measures is somewhat compromised. However, the above recommendations are prudent measures that should reduce the risk of acquiring and transmitting A.I.D.S.[1]

"Straights are more likely than gays to be closed-minded about A.I.D.S. The gay community is far more familiar with a wider variety of sex-related diseases than are straight people; this greater familiarity probably accounts for gays being more capable than straights of confronting a new sex-related disease like A.I.D.S. And it does seem that straight people have a particularly hard time coping with any sex-related disease.

Witness straight attitudes toward genital herpes simplex. This disease — often causing more discomfort than harm in straights, and easily preventable if people abstain from sex during their few days of active recurrence — has become the new 'leprosy' among straights.

Straights who don't have herpes live in terror of getting it; those who have it are filled with shame, cringing at every mention of the disease, every cheap, inaccurate joke, every 'horror' story printed in established newspapers or broadcast on television.

As a result, some straight people who have herpes are so afraid to let anyone know they have it that they will not even seek out information on the disease or speak to their physicians about the problem. What's worse, many straight herpes sufferers — either to avoid admitting their condition or out of anger at having contracted it — continue to have sex during periods of active recurrence, ensuring the spread of the disease. Thus, it can truly be said that genital herpes simplex is an epidemic fostered by ignorance, fear and shame.

As is apparent, straight attitudes about sex-related diseases have had a strong negative impact on the care of these diseases in the straight community. It is doubtful that these attitudes will do anything to help the gay community cope with the A.I.D.S. epidemic.

It seems apparent that changing straight atttudes about A.I.D.S. is not just a matter of improving public information about the disease. Without some changes in overall attitudes about sex-related diseases, many straights will find it hard to think clearly about any information they are given regarding A.I.D.S. To come to terms with A.I.D.S., straight people need to begin questioning their feelings about all sex-related disease. This, in turn, may mean a re-evaluation of basic attitudes about sex.

For example, isn't it possible that phobias about sex-related diseases are inspired by an underlying feeling that sex is 'dirty,' and that sex-related diseases are 'punishments' for sexual activity. This would account for feelings of shame surrounding sex-related diseases, as well as for feelings that A.I.D.S. is 'what you get' for a gay sexual lifestyle.

If so, the solution to the problem is clear. In informing the straight community about A.I.D.S., gay

38

people and straights sympathetic to gay issues need also to instill new perspectives on sex-related diseases and on sexuality in general.

This means structuring communications with an eye to several parameters: That A.I.D.S., and indeed all sex-related diseases, are first and foremost *illnesses* that need *treatment*; that myth and shame are the enemies of effective management of any epidemic — including epidemics of sex-related diseases. Ignorance and fear should not be allowed to prevent its treatment and encourage its spread."[2]

CHAPTER XIII FOOTNOTES

[1]Centers for Disease Control, *Morbidity and Mortality Weekly Report*, "Prevention of A.I.D.S."

[2]Dana Delibovi, "Straight Phobias About A.I.D.S.," *New York Native*, II, no. 26, (22 November - 5 December 1982), p. 10.

CHAPTER XIV
Possible Cures for
A.I.D.S.

"Doctors all over the country are experimenting with cures for A.I.D.S.; they have found that many of the infections, and even Kaposi's sarcoma, respond to medication up to a point. Pneumocystis pneumonia, for instance, can be treated with pentamidine, a drug that must be provided through the Centers for Disease Control. At several medical centers, scientists are treating Kaposi's sarcoma with some success. At New York University, 90 percent of treated patients have responded to VP 16-213 Etoposide, an experimental drug developed to treat leukemia and lymphoma.

At Memorial Sloan-Kettering Cancer Center in New York, Kaposi's sarcoma is being treated with the antiviral substance interferon. They are looking for an agent that might fight cancer, that might improve the immune system and that might have an antiviral effect.

Other efforts have also been made to reverse the underlying abnormality of A.I.D.S. Bone marrow transplants have been tried. Interferon and working with another byproduct of white blood cells called interleukin 2 has been tried. Experiments with different immune-stimulating drugs are being tried. The results are still being studied. But so far, it seems that the immune-system abnormalities of A.I.D.S. are almost always irreversible — at least by the time they are detected."[1]

"According to researchers at the Centers for Disease Control in Atlanta, the discovery of a hormone imbalance associated with A.I.D.S. could lead to a simple test that would reveal its presence quickly in patients and prevent its spread through blood transfusions.

The discovery also provides a hint that the disease might be caused by a recently identified human cancer virus.

According to a report presented March 7, 1983, at a meeting of the American Society for Microbiology in New Orleans, A.I.D.S. patients and people at risk for the disease have higher-than-normal levels of a hormone called thymosin alpha-1 in their bloodstreams.

Because the hormone can be measured with a simple blood test, it is possible that it could serve as an inexpensive way to identify people with A.I.D.S. or those likely to get it. It also could be used to detect the disease in blood donated for transfusion.

More research will be needed before measurement of the hormone can be used to spot the illness."[2]

"Behavioral changes are currently the only prudent advice physicians can offer. Some doctors hesitate to urge celibacy or monogamy on patients for whom casual sex is a way of life, but most seem to think the evidence is compelling enough to advocate just that.

One way to try to stop the syndrome from spreading further is to keep the A.I.D.S. agent out of the nation's blood supply if, indeed, a blood-borne virus is the culprit. Even that is still uncertain."[3]

CHAPTER XIV FOOTNOTES

[1]Henig, *New York Times Magazine*, p. 42.

[2]"Find Could Lead to Easy A.I.D.S. Test," *The Sacramento Bee (AP)*, (8 March 1983), p. A5.

[3]Henig, *New York Times Magazine*, p. 36.

CHAPTER XV
Treatment and Hospitalization of A.I.D.S. Victims

"Can A.I.D.S. be treated? There are no certain treatments at the present time for the varying degrees of immune deficiency that are seen in A.I.D.S. There are, however, treatments for individual episodes of the opportunistic infections, for Kaposi's sarcoma and for the other diseases to which A.I.D.S. predisposes. These treatments include antibiotics, chemotherapy, radiation therapy and experimental agents and techniques. Unfortunately, many of these treatments are transient in effect, costly, irregularly available and not without risks."[1]

"Treatment for A.I.D.S. must be approached in two ways: one is therapy for Kaposi's sarcoma and the infections themselves and the other is treatment that will try to repair the abnormalities of the immune system.

While there are treatments for the infections and even frequently effective chemotherapy for Kaposi's sarcoma, there is (so far) nothing that will cure — or even improve — the underlying immunologic dysfunction. Unfortunately, chemotherapy may further damage the immune system and its use is therefore justifiable only when Kaposi's sarcoma is immediately life-threatening. This is rarely the case. Despite the fear that is created by the diagnosis of a malignant tumor, people with Kaposi's sarcoma are seldom as ill as those who are first seen because of a serious opportunistic infection.

Obviously, the best approach would be any treatment that is directed at improving the function of the immune system. Both plasmapheresis and interferon have been discussed as means of achieving this end. Of these two approaches, there is a rational basis for using plasmapheresis, while a great deal of caution should accompany the use of interferon.

Plasma is the fluid in which the cellular elements of the blood are suspended. These cells include red and white blood cells. Lymphocytes are one type of white blood cell and an important component of the immune system.

Dissolved in the plasma are various substances including antibodies. Plasmapheresis is a procedure in which a quantity of blood is removed from the body and the cellular elements of the plasma are effectively retained. The procedure involves separating and returning only these cells to the patient, frequently in an albumen solution to replace the volume of plasma that has been withdrawn (see Appendix B).

The assumption underlying the treatment of A.I.D.S. victims is that their plasma contains injurious substances. There are (at least) two classes of substances that could impair the function of the immune system: Immune complexes, which are found in the blood of severely ill patients, and antibodies that may react with certain lymphocytes.

An immune complex is an aggregate of antibody molecules with or without the substance that stimulated the production of the antibodies in the first place. That substance is called an antigen; thus, the immune complex contains antigen in combination with its antibody.

Immune complexes are not normally found in the circulation, but they occur in the course of some diseases. While the presence of immune complexes in the bloodstream is not necessarily deleterious, their presence may correlate with the severity of the disease and they have been shown to cause tissue damage. They are most often associated with kidney ailments because they tend to be deposited in the kidneys. When immune complexes are found in the blood of cancer patients, the prognosis tends to be less favorable.

Because lymphocytes have receptors that bind immune complexes, immune complexes may interfere with the normal function of lymphocytes. It is certain, in any case, that immune complexes can do no good and it is not unreasonable to try to remove them from the bloodstream, particularly when dealing with an immune system that is already malfunctioning. Plasmapheresis has been shown to be of value in treating some patients who have immune complexes in their bloodstream — specifically, in treating certain patients with autoimmune diseases. An autoimmune disease is a disease in which ill effects occur because the body is producing antibodies directed against parts of the body itself. Manifestations of this ailment depend on which autoreactive antibody is produced. Sometimes, patients with A.I.D.S. produce auto-antibodies. For example, in the disease called autoimmune thrombocytopenia, the blood platelets (important in bloodclotting) are destroyed by antibodies that are produced against them. Apart from these anti-platelet antibodies it is not clear that the other antibodies that have been found in A.I.D.S. patients are necessarily harmful. There is, however, some evidence that some autoantibodies may indeed be reacting with some lymphocytes. These antibodies would also be removed by plasmapheresis.

The origin of the immune complexes in A.I.D.S. is unknown. Undoubtedly, there are several different antigens involved. One source that has absolutely been demonstrated is sperm. Because sperm and T-lymphocytes share certain components, sperm may also stimulate the production of antibodies that react against lymphocytes.

Sperm is also a major vehicle for the transmission of cytomegalovirus (CMV), which may be partly responsible for the immunological abnormalities discussed above. Patients with A.I.D.S. — as well as some healthy gay men — develop antibodies to sperm. Some of the healthy gay mean also have immune complexes in their circulation, and it is likely that sperm-related antigens in combination with their antibodies form at least part of the immune complexes in these cases. There have been similar findings among men who have been vasectomized.

Thus, sperm can act as an immunizing agent in the context of gay sex, a fact that in itself is clearly without harmful effects (A.I.D.S. is only a recent phenomenon among gay men). But sperm is not the only antigen associated with immune complexes, nor is it the only source of autoreactive antibodies in A.I.D.S.

It should be noted that sperm in the bloodstream of animals has been found to suppress the immune system.

Whatever their origin, both immune complexes and autoreactive antibodies can be removed by plasmapheresis. These, then, are the theoretical reasons for trying plasmapheresis in A.I.D.S. patients with immune complexes in their circulation. The procedure is not without some risk, but harm has only infrequently been caused. Certainly in the case of a fatal disease for which there are no established treatment options, it must be tried.

It is ironic that many gay men are plasmapheresed at weekly — sometimes twice weekly — intervals so that hepatitis B vaccine and hepatitis B antibody can be made from their plasma. In fact, these men are paid $50 per session. This program has been underway for some years and, thus far, there seem to be no harmful effects. It is, of course, possible that the gay men on this plasmapheresis program have been protected from A.I.D.S., a point that could be readily investigated by the New York Blood Center or other plasmapheresis centers.

Trials of interferon have been proposed as treatment for the underlying immunological disorder. Interferon is a highly potent substance which has both stimulating and inhibiting effects on the immune system. Since nobody knows what interferon will do, some feel that to propose its use in treating gay men with A.I.D.S. is to propose using gay men as guinea pigs.

There are abundant questions and comments in the interferon literature, many of them on the possibility that interferon may in fact mediate some of the damage that is seen in some autoimmune diseases. It also seems strange to propose the use of interferon in treating a disease in which interferon itself is frequently found in the blood of the patient. A distinctive type of interferon is produced by some patients with autoimmune diseases such as lupus. Patients with A.I.D.S. frequently have the same type of interferon in their blood. If this interferon is harmful in patients with lupus, the same is possible in patients with A.I.D.S. Certain abnormal structures can be seen in the lymphocytes of patients with some autoimmune diseases and similar structures have been detected in the lymphocytes of Kaposi's sarcoma patients. These 'tubulo reticular arrays,' as they are called, have been induced by exposure of cells to interferon."[2]

"In a recent study, out of 70 patients with Kaposi's sarcoma; 30 of them have received interferon. Of the 12 who completed the treatment before February 1982, three have no evidence of cancer and their immune function is improved; three have showed partial response; and six have shown no response. The remaining 18 have not completed their course of treatment.

There are many who feel that interferon might also be useful in the treatment of A.I.D.S. itself."[3]

"Certainly there is controversy surrounding the use of interferon. Many feel that this controversy should not be resolved by experimenting on gay men or on any other group.

One point that needs to be emphasized is that the use of interferon as an agent to effect changes in the immunologic function of a patient is not the same as using it as therapy for Kaposi's sarcoma. The trials that have already been undertaken with Kaposi's sarcoma patients will show if the opportunistic infections continue to occur in individuals whose Kaposi's sarcoma has responded to interferon treatment.

To be sure, the management of A.I.D.S. has been a learning experience for the doctors involved. They are dealing with an unfamiliar condition, and when the disease is not immediately life-threatening, they must be even more alert to the theoretical risks of untried treatments."[4]

The following excerpts are reprinted from an article by Larry Kramer in the *New York Native*, March 14-27 issue:

"It is very difficult for a patient to find out which hospital to go to or which doctor to go to or which mode of treatment to attempt.

Hospitals and doctors are reluctant to reveal how well they're doing with each type of treatment. They may, if you press them, give you a general idea. Most will not show you their precise numbers of how many patients are doing well on what and how many failed to adequately respond.

Because of the ludicrous requirements of the medical journals, doctors are prohibited from revealing publicly the specific data they are gathering from their treatments of our bodies. Doctors and hospitals need money for research and this money (from the National Institutes of Health, from rich patrons) comes based on the performance of their work (i.e., their tabulations of their results of their treatment of our bodies); this performance is written up as 'papers' that must be submitted to and accepted by such 'distinguished' medical publications as the *New England Journal of Medicine*. Most of these 'distinguished' publications, however, will not publish anything that has been spoken of, leaked, announced, or intimated publicly in advance. Even after acceptance, the doctors must hold their tongues until the article is actually published. Dr. Bijan Safai of Sloan-Kettering has been waiting for over six months for the *New England Journal*, which has accepted his interferon study, to publish it. Until that happens, he is only permitted to speak in the most general terms of how interferon is or is not working.

Priorities in this area appear to be peculiarly out of kilter at this extreme moment of life or death.

Let's talk about hospitals. Everybody's full, fellows. No room at the inn.

Part of this is simply overcrowding. Part of this is cruel.

Sloan-Kettering still enforces a regulation from pre-A.I.D.S. days that only one dermatology patient per week can be admitted to that hospital. (Kaposi's sarcoma falls under dermatology at Sloan-Kettering.) But Sloan-Kettering is also the second largest treatment center of A.I.D.S. patients in New York. You can be near to death and still not get into Sloan-Kettering.

Additionally, Sloan-Kettering (and the Food and Drug Administration) requires patients to receive their initial shots of interferon while they are hospitalized. A lot of men want to try interferon at Sloan-Kettering before trying chemotherapy elsewhere.

It's not hard to see why there's such a waiting time to get into Sloan-Kettering.

Most hospital staffs are still so badly educated about A.I.D.S. that they don't know much about it, except that they've heard it's contagious. Hence, A.I.D.S. patients are often treated as lepers."[5]

CHAPTER XV FOOTNOTES

[1] Mass, "Basic Questions," *New York Native*, pp. 23, 25.

[2] Joseph A. Sonnabend, M.D., "Treating the Epidemic," *New York Native*, III, no. 2, (20 December - 2 January 1983), p. 23.

[3] Henig, *New York Times Magazine*, p. 42.

[4] Sonnabend, *New York Native*.

[5] Kramer, *New York Native*, March 14-27.

CHAPTER XVI
Health Insurance and Welfare Problems of A.I.D.S. Victims

"Many of the ways of treating A.I.D.S. are experimental and many health insurance policies do not cover most of them.

Many serious victims of A.I.D.S. have been unable to qualify for welfare or disability or Social Security benefits. There are increasing numbers of men unable to work and unable to claim welfare because A.I.D.S. is not on the list of qualifying disability illnesses. (Immune deficiency is an acceptable determining factor for welfare among children, but not adults.) There are increasing numbers of men unable to pay their rent because of their illnesses and men with serious A.I.D.S. are being fired from certain jobs.

The stories in this area, of those suddenly found destitute, of those facing this illness with insufficient insurance, continue to mount."[1]

CHAPTER XVI FOOTNOTE

[1] Kramer, *New York Native.*

CHAPTER XVII
The Future Outlook
for A.I.D.S.

"Even after the agent causing A.I.D.S. is found, the spread of A.I.D.S. might still be impossible to stop. Like hepatitis B, the A.I.D.S. agent probably can be harbored for months before it causes problems. The incubation period for A.I.D.S. is thought to be at least six to eight months and could be as long as two years. This means that people who have already been infected might not know it until sometime between mid-1983 and the end of 1984. By then, each carrier might have unknowingly infected hundreds more individuals — through sexual contact, through blood donations, or through some yet unimagined route."[1]

Dr. Lawrence Mass, in his article, "The Case Against Medical Panic," in the *New York Native* stated:

"A.I.D.S. victims must avoid and discourage panic. Panic is not a constructive response to any crisis. At best, it is totally random, without direction or hope. A.I.D.S. has been described by federal health officials as. . . .

> *'perhaps the most serious epidemic of an apparently new infectious disease in this country since polio.'*

Like polio, however, A.I.D.S. will eventually be understood and controlled. As was the case with polio, behavioral approaches toward understanding and controlling A.I.D.S. are likely to be relatively ineffective. A major priority at this time is to discourage sexual lifestyles that involve many different, especially anonymous, partners. But the number one priority is to identify and eradicate the cause(s) of this disaster. While A.I.D.S. is very serious at this time and likely to become more so, in some segments of the population and in some locations more than others, it should be kept in the very broadest perspective that incomparably greater numbers of people will continue to die from traffic accidents and from cigarette and alcohol-related diseases.

Respect for the diversity and complexity of the issues that are involved is a must. Complex problems are not solved instantly or with simple solutions. The epidemic is not going to be fully understood or controlled in a matter of weeks or even moths. It's going to take years."[2]

CHAPTER XVII FOOTNOTES

[1] Henig, *New York Times Magazine*, p. 44.

[2] Lawrence Mass, M.D., "The Case Against Medical Panic," *New York Native*, III, no. 4, (17-30 January 1982), p. 25.

Author's Note: Current reports suggest that the incubation period may be as long as four years.

CHAPTER XVIII
Where to Go for Help

The Centers for Disease Control has identified A.I.D.S. cases in 34 states as well as 15 nations outside of the United States. The majority of cases are centered in the New York-New Jersey area, the San Francisco Bay Area, Los Angeles and Houston.

There is a National STD/VD Hotline (800) 227-8922 that will answer A.I.D.S. questions and provide referrals for help. Their hours are 9:00 a.m. to 9:00 p.m., California time. This organization is operated by the American Social Health Association and funded by the Centers for Disease Control, Atlanta, Georgia.

Following is a list of organizations that concerned individuals can contact in some of our major metropolitan areas about A.I.D.S.:

ATLANTA
A.I.D. Atlanta
P. O. Box 52785
Atlanta, GA 30305
(404) 872-0600 (A.I.D.S. Help Line)

BALTIMORE
Baltimore Gay Community Center
241-43 West Chase Street
Baltimore, MD 21201
(301) 837-2050

BOSTON
Boston Department of Health A.I.D.S. Hotline
(617) 414-5916

CHICAGO
Howard Brown Memorial Clinic
2676 North Halsted Street
Chicago, IL 60614
(312) 871-5777

DENVER
Gay and Lesbian Community Center
1436 Lafayette Street
Denver, CO 80218
(303) 831-6268

HOUSTON
Kaposi's Sarcoma Committee
3317 Montrose Boulevard
P.O. Box 1115
Houston, TX 77006
(800) 391-2040 (for those in Texas, except Houston)
(713) 792-3245 (for everyone else)

LOS ANGELES
KS Foundation/Los Angeles
1213 North Highland Avenue
Los Angeles, CA 90038
(213) 461-1333 (A.I.D.S. Hotline)

NEW YORK
National Gay Task Force
80 Fifth Avenue
New York, NY 10011
(800) 221-7044 (Nationwide Crisis line)
(212) 807-6016 (New York State only Crisis line)

PHILADELPHIA
A.I.D.S. Task Force
In care of PCHA
P.O. Box 7259
Philadelphia, PA 19101
(215) 232-8055 (PCHA Hotline)

SACRAMENTO
Kaposi's Sarcoma Foundation
2115 J Street
Suite 3
Sacramento, CA 95816
(916) 448-A.I.D.S.

SAN FRANCISCO
KS Research and Education Foundation, Inc.
520 Castro Street
P. O. Box 3360
San Francisco, CA 94114
(415) 864-4376 (A.I.D.S. Hotline)

WASHINGTON, D.C.
Whitman-Walker Health Clinic
2335 - 18th Street, N.W.
Washington, D.C. 20009
(202) 332-5295

LIST OF
WORKS CITED

Books

Marks, Geoffrey and William K. Beatty. *Epidemics*, NY: Scribners, 1976.

Articles and Periodicals

Amarnick, Claude, M.D. "Gay Physicians Respond to Criticism," *New York Native*, III, no. 1, (6-19 December 1982), 9.

Bush, Larry. "Reagan Playing Shell Games with A.I.D.S. Funding," *New York Native*, III, no. 6, (14-27 February 1983), 9, 10.

Callen, Michael, Richard Berkowitz, Richard Dworkin. "We Know Who We Are — Two Gay Men Declare War on Promiscuity," *New York Native*, II, no. 25, (8-21 November 1982), 25.

Delibovi, Dana. "Straight Phobias About A.I.D.S.," *New York Native*, II, no. 26, (22 November-5 December 1982), 10.

"Find Could Lead to Easy A.I.D.S. Test," *The Sacramento Bee*, (8 March 1983), A5.

Henig, Robin Marantz. "A.I.D.S. — A New Disease's Deadly Odyssey," *New York Times Magazine*, (6 February 1983), 28-31, 36, 38, 42, 44.

"House OKs Money for A.I.D.S. Study" *The Sacramento Union (AP)*, June 14, 1983, p. 1.

Kramer, Larry. "1,112 and Counting," *New York Native*, III, no. 8, (14-27 March 1983), 1, 15, 17, 18, 19, 21-23.

Mass, Lawrence M.D. "Basic Questions, Basic Answers About The Epidemic," *New York Native*, III, no. 3, (3-16 January 1983), 21-23, 25.

Mass, Lawrence M.D. "The Case Against Medical Panic," *New York Native*, III, no. 4, (17-30 January 1983), p. 25.

Mass, Lawrence M.D. "Congress Looks At the Epidemic," *New York Native*, II, no. 12, (10-23 May 1982), p. 17.

Mass, Lawrence M.D. "The Epidemic Continues," *New York Native*, II, no. 9, (29 March - 11 April 1982), p. 12.

Mass, Lawrence M.D. "Gays and Bad Blood: No Scapegoating — Yet," *New York Native*, III, no. 4, 17-30 January 1983), p. 8.

Seitzman, Peter A., M.D. "Guilt and A.I.D.S.," *New York Native*, III, no. 3, (3-16 January 1983), p. 23.

Sonnabend, Joseph A., M.D. "Treating The Epidemic," *New York Native*, III, no. 2, (20 December - 2 January 1983), pp. 21-23.

Stanley, Don. "A.I.D.S. Nightmare: Puzzling, Deadly — And Spreading," *The Sacramento Bee*, Scene, (4 January 1983), A18, col. 1-6, A19, col. 3, 4.

Stanley, Don. "A.I.D.S. The Price of Sex?", *The Sacramento Bee*, Scene, (1 March 1983), B5, col. 1-6, B7, col. 1-3.

Vachon, Ron. "If KS Had Hit Tennis Players," *New York Native*, II, no. 11, (26 April - 9 May 1982), p. 11.

West, Susan. "One Step Behind A Killer," *Science 83*, IV, no. 2, (March 1983), pp. 36-45.

Reports

Centers for Disease Control. "Prevention of Acquired Immune Deficiency Syndrome (A.I.D.S.): Report of Inter-Agency Recommendations," *Morbidity and Mortality Weekly Report*, XXXII, no. 8, (4 March 1983), pp. 101-103.

U. S. Department of Health and Human Services, Public Health Service/Centers for Disease Control. *"The Case Definition of A.I.D.S. Used by CDC for Epidemiologic Surveillance,"* Atlanta, 1-3.

U.S. Department of Health and Human Services, Public Health Service, Centers for Disease Control. *"Questions and Answers on Acquired Immune Deficiency Syndrome (A.I.D.S.),"* Atlanta, (November 1982).

U.S. Department of Health and Human Services, Public Health Service/Centers for Disease Control. *"Status of Acquired Immune Deficiency Syndrome (A.I.D.S.),"* Atlanta, (October 1, 1982).

Unpublished Material

Kaposi's Sarcoma Foundation. "Kaposi's Sarcoma and Other Diseases of the Acquired Immune Deficiency Syndrome," San Francisco.

Other Sources

Gonzales, Marty. "A.I.D.S.", TV News Documentary, KCRA-TV, Channel 3(Sacramento), 11:00 p.m. News, 23 March 1983.

NEW YORK

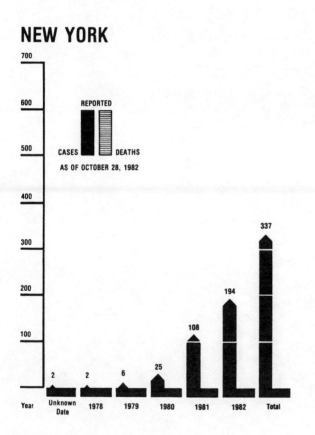

NEW YORK = 337

UNITED STATES

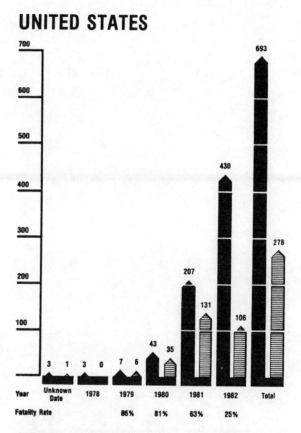

TOTAL CASES: U.S. = 693

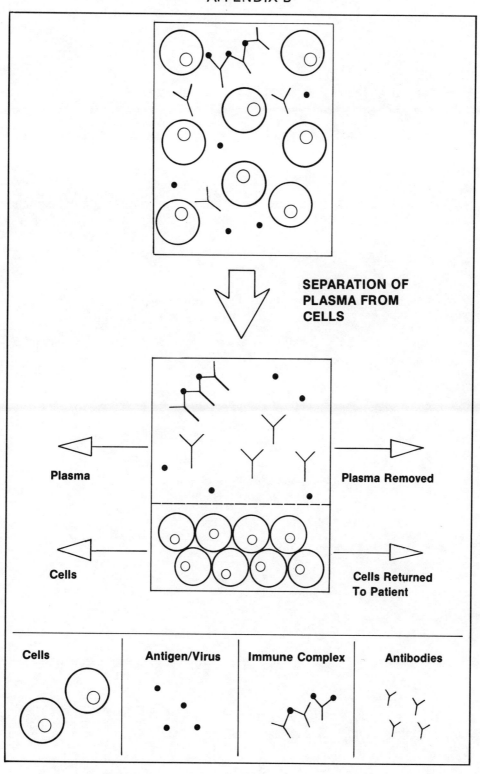

SEPARATION OF
PLASMA FROM
CELLS

Plasma

Plasma Removed

Cells

Cells Returned
To Patient

| Cells | Antigen/Virus | Immune Complex | Antibodies |

APPENDIX C

MEDICAL HISTORY AND DATA PERTAINING TO A.I.D.S. AND A.I.D.S.-RELATED
DISEASES WITH INDIVIDUAL CASE HISTORIES

Reprinted from the *Morbidity and Mortality Weekly* Report

June 5, 1981

Pneumocystis Pneumonia — Los Angeles

In the period October 1980-May 1981, 5 young men, all active homosexuals, were treated for biopsy-confirmed Pneumocystis carinii pneumonia at 3 different hospitals in Los Angeles, California. Two of the patients died. All 5 patients had laboratory-confirmed previous or current cytomegalovirus (CMV) infection and candidal mucosal infection. Case reports of these patients follow.

Patient 1: A previously healthy 33-year-old man developed P. carinii pneumonia and oral mucosal candidiasis in March 1981 after a 2-month history of fever associated with elevated liver enzymes, leukopenia, and CMV viruria. The serum complement-fixation CMV titer in October 1980 was 256; in May 1981 it was 32.* The patient's condition deteriorated despite courses of treatment with trimethoprim-sulfamethoxazole (TMP/SMX), pentamidine, and acyclovir. He died May 3, and postmortem examination showed residual P. carinii and CMV pneumonia, but no evidence of neoplasia.

Patient 2: A previously healthy 30-year-old man developed P. carinii pneumonia in April 1981 after a 5-month history of fever each day and of elevated liver-function tests, CMV viruria, and documented seroconversion to CMV, i.e., an acutephase titer of 16 and a convales-cent-phase titer of 28* in anticomplement immunofluorescence tests. Other features of his illness included leukopenia and mucosal candi-diasis. His pneumonia responded to a course of intravenous TMP/SMX, but, as of the latest reports, he continues to have a fever each day.

Patient 3: A 30-year-old man was well until January 1981 when he developed esophageal and oral candidiasis that responded to Am-photericin B treatment. He was hospitalized in February 1981 for P. carinii pneumonia that responded to oral TMP/SMX. His esophageal candidiasis recurred after the pneumonia was diagnosed, and he was again given Amphotericin B. The CMV complement-fixation titer in March 1981 was 8. Material from an esophageal biopsy was positive for CMV.

Patient 4: A 29-year-old man developed P. carinii pneumonia in February 1981. He had had Hodgkins disease 3 years earlier, but had been successfully treated with radiation therapy alone. He did not improve after being given intravenous TMP/SMX and corticosteroids and died in March. Postmortem examination showed no evidence of Hodgkins disease, but P. carinii and CMV were found in lung tissue.

Patient 5: A previously healthy 36-year-old man with a clinical diagnosed CMV infection in September 1980 was seen in April 1981 because of a 4-month history of fever, dyspnea, and cough. On admission he was found to have P. carinii pneumonia, oral candidiasis, and CMV retinitis. A complement-fixation CMV titer in April 1981 was 128. The patient has been treated with 2 short courses of TMP/SMX that have been limited because of a sulfa-induced neutropenia. He is being treated for candidiasis with topical nystatin.

The diagnosis of Pneumocystis pneumonia was confirmed for all 5 patients antemortem by closed or open lung biopsy. The patients did not know each other and had no known common contacts or knowledge of sexual partners who had had similar illnesses. The 5 did not have comparable histories of sexually transmitted disease. Four had serologic evidence of past hepatitis B infection but had no evidence of current hepatitis B surface antigen. Two of the 5 reported having frequent homosexual contacts with various partners. All 5 reported using inhalant drugs, and 1 reported parenteral drug abuse. Three patients had profoundly depressed numbers of thymus-dependent lymphocyte cells and profoundly depressed in vitro proliferative responses to mitogens and antigens. Lymphocyte studies were not performed on the other 2 patients.

Reported by MS Gottlieb, MD, HM Schanker, MD, PT Fan, MD, A Saxon, MD, JD Weisman, DO, Div. of Clinical Immunology-Allergy, Dept of Medicine, UCLA School of Medicine; I Pozalski, MD, Cedars-Mt. Sinai Hospital, Los Angeles; Field Services Div, Epidemiology Program Office, CDC.

Editorial Note: Pneumocystis pneumonia in the United States is almost exclusively limited to severely immunosuppressed patients(1). The occurrence of pneumocystosis in these 5 previously healthy individuals without a clinically apparent underlying immunodeficiency is unusual. The fact that these patients were all homosexuals suggests an association between some aspect of a homosexual lifestyle or disease acquired through sexual contact and Pneumocystis pneumonia in this population. All 5 patients described in this report has laboratory-confirmed CMV disease or virus shedding within 5 months of the diagnosis of Pneumocystis pneumonia. CMV infection has been shown to induce transient abnormalities of in vitro cellularimmune function in otherwise healthy human hosts(2,3). Although all 3 patients tested had abnormal cel-lular-immune function, no definitive conclusion regarding the role of CMV infection in these 5 cases can be reached because of the lack of published data on cellular-immune function in healthy homosexual males with and without CMV antibody. In 1 report, 7 (3.6%) of 194 patients with pneumocystosis also had CMV infection; 40 (21%) of the same group had at least 1 other major concurrent infection(1). A high prevalence of CMV infections among homosexual males was recently reported: 179 (94%) of 190 males reported to be exclusively homosex-ual had serum antibody to CMV, and 14 (7.4%) has CMV viruria; rates for 101 controls of similar age who were reported to be exclusively heterosexual were 54% for seropositivity and zero for viruria(4). In another study of 64 males, 4 (6.3%) had positive tests for CMV in semen, but none had CMV recovered from urine. Two of the 4 reported recent homosexual contacts. These findings suggest not only that virus shedding may be more readily detected in seminal fluid than in urine, but alsothat seminal fluid may be an important vehicle of CMV trans-mission(5).

All of the above observations suggest the possibility of a cellular-immune dysfunction related to a common exposure that predisposes individuals to opportunistic infections such as pneumocystosis and candidiasis. Although the role of CMV infection in the pathogenesis of pneumocystosis remains unknown, the possibility of P. carinii infection must be carefully considered in a differential diagnosis for previously

---

*Paired specimens not run in parallel.

healthy homosexual males with dyspnea and pneumonia.

References

1. Walzer PD, Perl DP, Krogstad DJ, Rayson PG, Schultz MG. Pneumocystis carinii pneumonia in the United States. Epidemiologic, diagnostic, and clinical features. Ann Intern Med 1974; 80:83-93.
2. Rinaldo CR, Jr, Black PH, Hirsch MS. Interaction of cytomegalovirus with leukocytes from patients with mononucleosis due to cytomegalovirus. J Infec Dis 1977;136:667-78.
3. Rinaldo CR, Jr. Carney WP, Richter BS, Black PH, Hirsch MS. Mechanisms of immunosuppression in cytomegaloviral mononucleosis. J Infect Dis 1980;141:488-95.
4. Drew WL, Mintz L, Miner RC, Sands M, Ketterer B. Prevalence of cytomegalovirus infection in homosexual men. J Infect Dis 1981; 143:188-92.
5. Lang DJ, Kummer JF. Cytomegalovirus in semen: observations in selected populations. J Infect Dis 1975,132:472-3.

July 3, 1981

Kaposi's Sarcoma and Pneumocystis Pneumonia Among Homosexual Men — New York City and California

During the past 30 months, Kaposi's sarcoma (KS), an uncommonly reported malignancy in the United States, has been diagnosed in 26 homosexual men (20 in New York City [NYC]; 6 in California). The 26 patients range in age from 26-51 years (mean 39 years). Eight of these patients died (7 in NYC, 1 in California)—all 8 within 24 months after KS was diagnosed. The diagnoses in all 26 cases were based on histopathological examination of skin lesions, lymph nodes, or tumor in other organs. Twenty-five of the 26 patients were white, 1 was black. Presenting complains from 20 of these patients are shown in Table 1.

TABLE 1. Presenting complaints in 20 patients with Kaposi's sarcoma

Presenting complaint	Number (percentage) of patients
Skin lesion(s) only	10 (50%)
Skin lesions plus lymphadenopathy	4 (20%)
Oral mucosal lesion only	1 (5%)
Inguinal adenopathy plus perirectal abscess	1 (5%)
Weight loss and fever	2 (10%)
Weight loss, fever and pneumonia (one due to Pneumocystis carinii)	2 (10%)

Skin or mucous membrane lesions, often dark blue to violaceous plaques or nodules, were present in most of the patients on their initial physician visit. However, these lesions were not always present and often were considered benign by the patient and his physician.

A review of the New York University Coordinated Cancer Registry for KS in men under age 50 revealed no cases from 1970-1979 at Belevue Hospital and 3 cases in this age group at the New York University Hospital from 1961-1979.

Seven KS patients had serious infections diagnosed after their initial physician visit. Six patients has pneumonia (4 biopsy confirmed as due to Pneumocystis carinii [PC]), and one had necrotizing toxoplasmosis of the central nervous system. One of the patients with Pneumocystis pneumonia also experienced severe, recurrent, herpes simplex infection; extensive candidiasis; and cryptococcal meningitis. The results of tests for cytomegalovirus (CMV) infection were available for 12 patients. All 12 has serological evidence of past or present CMV infection. In 3 patients for whom culture results were available, CMV was isolated from blood, urine and/or lung of all 3. Past infections with amebiasis and hepatitis were commonly reported.

Since the previous report of 5 cases of Pneumocystis pneumonia in homosexual men from Los Angeles(1), 10 additional cases (4 in Los Angeles and 6 in the San Francisco Bay area) of biopsy-confirmed PC pneumonia have been identified in homosexual men in the state. Two of the 10 patients also have KS. This brings the total number of Pneumocystis cases among homosexual men in California to 15 since September 1979. Patients range in age from 25 to 46 years.

Reported by A Friedman-Kien, MD, L Laubenstein, MD, M Marmor, PhD, K Hymes, MD, J Green, MD, A Ragaz, MD, J Gottleib, MD, F Muggia, MD, R Demopoulos, MD, M Weintraub, MD, D Williams, MD, New York University Medical Center, NYC; R Oliveri, MD, J Marmer, MD, NYC; J Wallace, MD, I Halperin, MD, JF Gillooley, MD, St. Vincent's Hospital and Medical Center, NYC; N Prose, MD, Downstate Medical Center, NYC; E Klein, MD, Roosevelt Hospital, NYC; J Vogel, MD, B Safai, MD, P Myskowski, MD, C Urmacher, MD, B Koziner, MD, L Nisce, MD, M Kris, MD, D Armstrong, MD, J Gold, MD, Sloan-Kettering Memorial Institute, NYC; D Mildran, MD, Beth Israel Hospital, NYC; M Tapper, MD, Lenon Hill Hospital, NYC; JB Weissman, MD, Columbia Presbyterian Hospital, NYC; R Rothenberg, MD, State Epidemiologist, New York State Dept of Health; SM Friedman, MD, Acting Director, Bur of Preventable Diseases, New York City Dept of Health; FP Siegal, MD, Dept of Medicine, Mount Sinai School of Medicine, City College of New York, NYC; J Groundwater, MD, J Gilmore, MD, San Francisco; D Coleman, MD, S Follansbee, MD, J Gullett, MD, SJ Stegman, MD, University of California at San Francisco; C Wofsy, MD, San Francisco General Hospital, San Francisco; D Bush, MD, Franklin Hospital, San Francisco; L Drew, MD, PhD, Mt. Zion Hospital, E Braff, MD, S Dritz, MD, City/County Health Dept, San Francisco; M Klein, MD, Valley Memorial Hospital, Salinas; JK Preiksaitis, MD, Stanford University Medical Center, Palo Alto; MS Gottlieb, MD, University of California at Los Angeles; R Jung, MD, University of Southern California Medical Center, Los Angeles; J Chin, MD, State Epidemiologist, California Dept. of Health Services; J Goedert, MD, National Cancer Institute, National Institute of Health; Parasitic Diseases Div, Center for Infectious Diseases, VD Control Division, Center for Prevention Services, Chronic Diseases Div, Center for Envonmental Health, CDC.

Editorial Note: KS is a malignant neoplasm manifested primarily by multiple vascular nodules in the skin and other organs. The disease is multifocal, with a course ranging from indolent, with only skin manifestations, to fulminant, with extensive visceral involvement(2).

Accurate incidence and mortality rates for KS are not available for the United States, but the annual incidence has been estimated between 0.02-0.06 per 100,000; it affects primarily elderly males(3,4). In a series of 92 patients treated between 1949 and 1975 at the Memorial Sloan-Kettering Cancer Institute in NYC, 76% were male, and the mean age was 63 years (range 23-90 years) at the time of diagnosis(5).

The disease in elderly men is usually manifested by skin lesions and a chronic clinical course (mean survival time is 8-13 years)(2). Two exceptions to this epidemiologic pattern have been noted previously. The first occurs in an endemic belt across equatorial Africa, where KS commonly affects children and young adults and accounts for up to 9% of all cancers(3). Secondly, the disease appears to have a higher incidence in renal transplant recipients(6-9) and in others receiving immunosuppressive therapy(10-12).

The occurrence of this number of KS cases during a 30-month period among young, homosexual men is considered highly unusual. No previous association between KS and sexual preference has been reported. The fulminant clinical course reported in many of these patients also differs from that classically described for elderly persons.

The histopathologic diagnosis of KS may be difficult for 2 reasons. Changes in some lesions may be interpreted as nonspecific, and other cutaneous and soft tissue sarcomas, such as angiosarcoma of the skin, may be confused with KS(13,14).

That 10 new cases of Pneumocystis pneumonia have been identified in homosexual men suggests that the 5 previously reported cases were not an isolated phenomenon(1). In addition, CDC has a report of 4 homosexual men in NYC who developed severe, progressive, perianal herpes simplex infections and had evidence of cellular immunodeficiencies. Three died, 1 with systemic CMV infection. The fourth patient is currently undergoing therapy. It is not clear if or how the clustering of KS, pneumocystis, and other serious diseases in homosexual men is related. What is known is that the patients with Pneumocystis pneumonia described in the previous report showed evidence of impaired cellular immunity and previous or current CMV infection(1). Furthermore, serologic evidence of past CMV infection and active shedding of CMV have been shown to be much more common among homosexual men than heterosexual men attending a sexually transmitted disease clinic(15). A specific serologic association with CMV infection has been demostrated among American and European patients with KS(16,17) and herpes-type virus particles have been demonstrated in tissue culture cell lines from African cases of KS(18). It has been hypothesized that activation of oncogenic virus during periods of immunosuppression may result in the development of KS(19). Although immunosuppression often results in CMV infection, it is not yet clear whether CMV infection precedes or follows the above-mentioned disorders.

Although it is not certain that the increase in KS and PC pneumonia is restricted to homosexual men, the vast majority of recent cases have been reported from this group. Physicians should be alert for Kaposi's sarcoma, PC pneumonia, and other opportunistic infections associated with immunosuppression in homosexual men.

References

1. CDC. Pneumocystis pneumonia — Los Angeles. MMWR 1981; 30:250.
2. Safai B, Good RA. Kaposi's sarcoma: a review and recent developments. CA 1981;31:1-12.
3. Oettle AG. Geographical and racial differences in the frequency of Kaposi's sarcoma as evidence of environmental or genetic causes. Acta Un Int Cancr 1962;18:330-63.
4. Rothman S. Remarks on sex, age, and racial distribution of Kaposi's sarcoma and on possible pathogenetic factors. Acta Un Int Cancr 1962;18:326-9.
5. Safai B, Mike V, Giraldo G, Beth E, Good RA. Association of Kaposi's sarcoma with second primary malignancies: possible etiopathogenic implications. Cancer 1980;45:1472-9.
6. Harewood AR, Osoba D, Hofstader SL, et al. Kaposi's sarcoma in recipients of renal transplants. Am J Med 1979;67:759-65.
7. Stibling J, Weitzner S, Smith GV: Kaposi sarcoma in renal allograft recipients. Cancer 1978;42:442-6.
8. Myers BD, Kessler E, Levi J, Pick A, Rosenfeld JB, Tikvah P. Kaposi sarcoma in kidney transplant recipients. Arch Intern Med 1974; 133:307-11.
9. Penn I. Kaposi's sarcoma in organ transplant recipients: report of 20 cases. Transplantation 1979;27:8-11.
10. Gange RW, Jones EW. Kaposi's sarcoma and immunosuppressive therapy: an appraisal. Clin Exp Dermatol 1978;3:135-46.
11. Klepp O, Dahl O, Stenwig JT. Association of Kaposi's sarcoma and prior immunosuppressive therapy: a 5-year material of Kaposi's sarcoma in Norway. Cancer 1978;42:2626-30.
12. Hoshaw RA, Schwartz RA. Kaposi's sarcoma after immunosuppressive therapy with prednisone. Arch Dermatol 1980;116:1280-2.
13. Girard C, Johnson WC, Graham JH. Cutaneous angiosarcoma. Cancer 1970;26:868-83.

14. Rosai J, Sumner HW, Kostianovsky M, Perez-Mesa C. Angiosarcoma of the skin. A clinicopathologic and fine structural study. Hum Pathol 1976;7:83-109.

15. Drew WL, Mintz L, Miner RC, Sands M, Ketterer B. Prevalence of cytomegalovirus infection in homosexual men. J Infec Dis 1981; 143:188-92.

16. Giraldo G, Beth E, Kourilsky FM, et al. Antibody patterns of herpesvirus in Kaposi's sarcoma: serologic association of European Kaposi's sarcoma with cytomegalovirus. Int J Cancer 1975;15:839-48.

17. Giraldo G, Beth E, Henie W, et al. Antibody patterns to herpesvirus in Kaposi's sarcoma. II. serological association of American Kaposi's sarcoma with cytomegalovirus. Int J Cancer 1978;22:126-31.

18. Giraldo G, Beth E, Haguenau F. Herpes-type virus particles in tissue culture of Kaposi's sarcoma from different geogrphic regions. J Natl Cancer Inst 1972;49:1509-26.

19. Kapadia SB, Krause JR. Kaposi's sarcoma after long-term alkylating agent therapy for multiple myeloma. South Med J 1977;70: 1011-3.

August 28, 1981

Follow-Up on Kaposi's Sarcoma and Pneumocystis Pneumonia

Twenty-six cases of Kaposi's sarcoma (KS) and 15 cases of Pneumocystis carinii pneumonia (PCP) among previously healthy homosexual men were recently reported(1,2). Since July 3, 1981, CDC has received reports of an additional 70 cases of these 2 conditions in persons without known underlying disease. The sex, race, sexual preference, and mortality data known for 108 persons with either or both conditions are summarized in Table 1.

TABLE 1. Cases of Kaposi's sarcoma (KS) and Pneumocystis carinii pneumonia (PCP) reported to CDC with dates on onset between January 1976 and July 1981

Diagnosis (number of patients	Sex		Race of Men				Sexual preference of men			Fatality (percentage)
	Male	Female	White	Black	Hispanic	Unknown	Homosexual or bisexual	Heterosexual	Unknown	
KS and PCP (N=7)	7	0	5	0	1	1	7	0	0	3/7 (43%)
KS only (N=47)	47	0	41	3	3	0	44	1	2	8/47 (17%)
PCP only (N=54)	53	1	33	9	7	4	44	5	4	32/54 (59%)
Total (N=108)	107	1	79	12	11	5	95	6	6	43/108 (40%)

The majority of the reported cases of KS and/or PCP have occurred in white men. Patients ranged in age from 15-52 years; over 95% were men 25-49 years of age. Ninety-four percent (95/101) of the men for whom sexual preference was known were homosexual or bisexual. Forty percent of the reported cases were fatal. Of the 82 cases for which the month of diagnosis is known, 75 (91%) have occurred since January 1980, with 55 (67%) diagnosed from January through July 1981. Although physicians from several states have reported cases of KS and PCP among previously healthy homosexual men, the majority of cases have been reported from New York and California.

Reported by SM Friedman, MD, YM Feiman, MD, New York City Dept of Health; R Rothenberg, MD, State Epidemiologist, New York State Dept of Health; S Dritz, MD, E Braff, MD, City/County Health Dept, San Francisco; S Fannin, MD, Los Angeles County Dept of Health Svcs; I Heindl, MD, California Dept of Health Svcs; RK Sikes, DVM, State Epidemiologist, Georgia Dept of Human Resources; RA Gunn, MD, State Epidemiologist, Florida State Dept of Health and Rehabilitative Svcs; MA Roberts, PhD, State Epidemiologist, Oklahoma State Dept of Health; Task Force on Kaposi's Sarcoma and Opportunistic Infections, Center for Prevention Svcs, Center for Infectious Diseases, Center for Environmental Health, Field Svcs Div, Consolidated Surveillance and Communications Activities, Epidemiology Program Office, CDC.

Editorial Note: KS is a rare, malignant neoplasm seen predominantly in elderly men in this country. In eldermen men the disease is manifested by skin lesions and a chronic clinical course; it is rarely fatal(3). In contrast, the persons currently reported to have KS are young to middle-aged men, and 20% of the cases have been fatal. Although some of the patients have presented with a violaceous skin or mucous membrane lesions typical of KS, many such lesions have been initially overlooked. Other patients have been diagnosed by lymph-node biopsy after a prodrome consisting of fever, weight loss, and lymphadenopathy. Seven (13%) of fifty-four KS patients also had PCP. In many cases the histopathologic diagnosis from skin, lymph node, or visceral-lesion tissue has been difficult even in specialized hands.

The occurrence of Pneumocystis carinii pneumonia in patients who are not immunosuppressed due to known underlying disease or therapy is also highly unusual(4). Although 7(11%) of the 61 patients with PCP also had KS, in many instances pneumonia preceded the tumor. Although most of the patients with PCP reported recent respiratory symptoms, some gave a history of weeks to months of systemic symptoms including weight loss and general malais, similar to the prodrome described by patients who developed lymphadenopathic KS. Several of the patients with PCP has other serious infections, including gastrointestinal candidiasis, cryptococcal meningitis, and disseminated infections with Mycobacteriaceae and herpes simplex. Many of the PCP and KS patients have had positive cultures or serologic evidence of infection with cytomegalovirus.

The apparent clustering of both Pneumocystis carinii pneumonia and KS among homosexual men suggests a common underlying factor. Both diseases have been associated with host immunosuppression(4-6), and studies in progress are showing immunosuppression in some of these cases. The extent or cause of immune suppression is not known. Physicians should be aware of the possible occurrence of these diseases and other opportunistic infections, particularly among men with symptoms suggestive of these disorders or their prodromes, since therapy is specific and verification of the diagnosis requires biopsy.

Several state and local health departments and CDC are conducting active surveillance for KS, PCP, and opportunistic infections in persons without known predisposing underlying disease. A national case-control study will be implemented shortly.

References

1. CDC. Pneumocystis pneumonia — Los Angeles. MMWR 1981;30:250-2.
2. CDC. Kaposi's sarcoma and Pneumocystis pneumonia among homosexual men — New York City and California. MMWR 1981;30: 305-8.
3. Safai B, Good RA. Kaposi's sarcoma: a review and recent developments. CA 1981;31:1-12.
4. Walzer PD, Perl DP, Krogstad DJ, Rawsom PG, Schultz MG. Pneumocystis carinii pneumonia in the United States. Apidemiologic, diagnostic, and clinical features. Ann Intern Med 1974;80:83-93.
5. Penn I. Kaposi's sarcoma in organ transplant recipients: report of 20 cases. Transplantation 1979;27:8-11.
6. Gange RW, Jones EW. Kaposi's sarcoma and immunosuppressive therapy: an appraisal. Clin Exp Dermatol 1978;3:135-46.

May 21, 1982

Persistent, Generalized Lymphadenopathy among Homosexual Males

Since October 1981, cases of persistent, generalized lymphadenopathy — not attributable to previously identified causes — among homosexual males have been reported to CDC by physicians in several major metropolitan areas in the United States. These reports were prompted by an awareness generated by ongoing CDC and state investigations of other emerging health problems among homosexual males(1).

In February and March 1982, records were reviewed for 57 homosexual men with lymphadenopathy seen at medical centers in Atlanta, New York City, and San Francisco. The cases reviewed met the following criteria: 1) lymphadenopathy of at least 3 months' duration, involving 2 or more extra-inguinal sites, and confirmed on physical examination by the patient's physician; 2) absence of any current illness or drug use known to cause lymphadenopathy; and 3) presence of reactive hyperplasia in a lymph node, if a biopsy was performed.

The 57 patients had a mean age of 33 years and the following characteristics: all were male; 81% were white, 15% black, and 4% Hispanic; 83% were single, 6% married and 11% divorced; 86% were homosexual, 14% bisexual. The median duration of lymphadenopathy was 11 months. Ninety-five percent of patients had at least 3 node chains involved (usually cervical, axillary, and inguinal). Forty-three patients had had lymph node biopsies showing reactive hyperplasia. Approximately 70% of the patients had some constitutional symptoms including fatigue, 70%; fever, 49%; night sweats, 44%; and weight loss greater than or equal to 5 pounds, 28%. Hepatomegaly and/or splenomegaly was noted among 26% of patients.

Recorded medical histories for the 57 patients suggested that the use of drugs such as nitrite inhalants, marijuana, hallucinogens and cocaine was common. Many of these patients have a history of sexually transmitted infections (gonorrhea 58%, symphilis 47%, and amebiasis 42%). Of 30 patients skin-tested for delayed hypersensitivity response, 8 were found to be anergic on the basis of at least 2 antigens other than purified protein derivative (PPD).

Immunologic evaluation performed at CDC for 8 of the above patients demostrated abnormal T-lymphocyte helper-to-suppressor ratios (less than 0.9) for 2 patients. Since this review, immunologic evaluations at CDC of 13 additional homosexual males with lymphadenopathy from Atlanta and San Francisco revealed 6 with ratios of less than 0.9. The normal range of T-lymphocyte helper-to-suppressor ratios established in the CDC laboratory for healthy heterosexual patients is 0.9-3.5 (mean of 2.3). The normal range is being established for apparently healthy homosexual males.

Since the initiation of this study, 1 patient with lymphadenopathy has developed Kaposi's sarcoma.

Reported by D Mildvan, MD, U Mathur, MD, Div of Infectious Diseases, Beth Israel Medical Center, R Enlow, MD, Rheumatology Dept, Hospital for Joint Diseases, D Armstrong, MD, J Gold, MD, C Sears, MD, B Wong, MD, AE Brown, MD, S Henry, MD, Div of Infectious Disease, B Safai, MD, Dermatology Svc. Dept of Medicine, Z Arlin, MD, Div of Hematology, Memorial Sloan-Kettering Medical Center, A Moore, MD, C Metroka, MD, Div of Hematology-Oncology, L Drusin, MD, MPH, Dept of Medicine, The New York Hospital-Cornell Medical Center, I Spigland, MD, Div of Virology, Montefiore Hospital and Medical Center, DC William, MD, St Luke's-Roosevelt Hospital Center, F Siegal, MD, Dept of Medicine, J Brown, MD, Dept of Neoplastic Diseases, Mt. Sinai Medical Center, J Wallace, MD, Dept of Medicine, St. Vincent's Hospital and Medical Center, D Senser, MD, SM Friedman, MD, YM Felman, MD, New York City Dept of Health, R Rothenberg, MD, State Epidemiologist, New York State Dept of Health; RK Sikes, DVM, State Epidemiologist, Georgia Dept of Human Resources; W Owen, MD, Bay Area Physicians for Human Rights, S Dritz, MD, C Rendon, Bureau of Communicable Disease Control, San Francisco Dept of Public Health, J Chin, MD, State Epidemiologist, California Dept of Health Svcs; J Sonnabend, MD, Uniformed Svcs University of Health Sciences, Bethesda, E Israel, MD, State Epidemiologist, Maryland State Dept of Health and Mental Hygiene; Special Studies Br, Center for Environmental Health, Div of Viral Diseases, Div of Host Factors, Center for Infectious Diseases, Field Svcs Div, Epidemiology Program Office, Task Force on Kaposi's Sarcoma and Opportunistic Infections, Office of the Centers Director, CDC.

Editorial Note: The report above documents the occurrence of cases of unexplained, persistent, generalized lymphadenopathy among homosexual males. There are many known causes of generalized lymphadenopathy including viral infections (e.g., hepatitis B, infectious mononucleosis, cytomegalovirus infection, rubella), tuberculosis, disseminated Mycobacterium avium-intracellulare, syphilis, other bacterial and fungal infections, toxoplasmosis, connective tissue disorders, hypersensitivity drug reactions, heroin use, and neoplastic diseases (including leukemia and lymphoma)(2). Causes for the persistent lymphadenopathy among patients discussed above were sought but could not be identified.

This unexplained syndrome is of concern because of current reports of Kaposi's sarcoma (KS) and opportunistic infections (OI) that primarily involve homosexual males(1,3). Epidemiologic characteristics (age, racial composition, city of residence) of the homosexual patients with lymphadenopathy discussed here are similar to those of the homosexual KS/OI patients. Thirty-two (44%) of 73 Kaposi's sarcoma patients and 14 (23%) of 61 Pneumocystis carinii pneumonia patients reported to CDC in the period mid-June 1981-January 1982 had a history of lymphadenopathy before diagnosis(3). Mycobacterium avium-intracellulare (an opportunistic agent) has been isolated from the lymph nodes of a homosexual patient(4). Moreover, the findings of anergy and depressed T-lymphocyte helper-to-suppressor ratios in some of the patients with lymphadenopathy suggest cellular immune dysfunction. Patients with KS/OI have had severe abnormalities of cellular immunity (5,6). The relationship between immunologic findings for patients with lymphadenopathy and patients with KS/OI remains to be determined.

Although these cases have been identified and defined on the basis of the presence of lymphadenopathy, this finding may be merely a manifestation of an underlying immunologic or other disorder that needs to be characterized further. Virologic and immunologic studies of many of these patients are currently under way. An analysis of trends in incidence for lymphadenopathy over the past several years is being conducted to determine whether this syndrome is new and whether homosexual males are particularly affected. Results of these studies and follow-up of these patients are necessary before the clinical and epidemiologic significance of persistent, generalized lymphadenopathy among homosexual males can be determined. Homosexual males patients with unexplained, persistent, generalized lymphadenopathy should be followed for periodic review.

References

1. CDC. Kaposi's sarcoma and Pneumocystis pneumonia among homosexual men — New York City and California. MMWR 1981;30: 305-8.
2. Wintrobe MM. Clinical hematology. 8th ed. Philadelphia: Lea and Febiger, 1981:1279-81.
3. CDC. Task Force on Kaposi's Sarcoma and Opportunistic Infections. Epidemiologic aspects of the current outbreak of Kaposi's sarcoma and opportunistic infections. N Engl J Med 1982;306:248-52.
4. Fainstein, V, Bolivar R, Mavligit G, Rios A, Luna M. Disseminated infection due to Mycobacterium avium-intracellulare in a homosexual man with Kaposi's sarcoma. J Infect Dis 1982;145:586.
5. Gottlieb M. Schroff R, Schanker H, et al. Pneumocystis carinii pneumonia and mucosal candidiasis in previously healthy homosexual men. N Engl J Med 1981;305:1425-31.
6. Masur H, Michelis MA, Greene JB, et al. An outbreak of community-acquired Pneumocystis carinii pneumonia: Initial manifestation of cellular immune dysfunction. N Engl J Med 1981;305:1431-8.

June 4, 1982

Diffuse, Undifferentiated Non-Hodgkins Lymphoma among Homosexual Males — United States

A recent outbreak of Kaposi's sarcoma, Pneumocystis carinii pneumonia, and other opportunistic infections (KSOI) involving homosexual males and associated with an acquired cellular immunodeficiency syndrome has been described(1,2). While the pathogenesis of these disorders among homosexual males in San Francisco was being studied, 4 cases of diffuse, undifferentiated non-Hodgkins lymphoma (DUNHL) were diagnosed between March 1981 and January 1982. Because of the rarity of this malignancy and the potential relationship of these cases to the KSOI syndrome, they are reported here.

Patient 1: A 28-year-old hospital clerk complained of back and shoulder pain starting in early March 1981. Within a few days he had swelling of the right eye and an unsteady gait, and he was hospitalized on March 21. "Shotty" peripheral lymphadenopathy was present. A biopsy of an orbital mass and an enlarged cervical lymph node disclosed DUNHL. A myelogram revealed a T4-T6 block by an extradural mass. Radiation and chemotherapy led to complete remission. In September 1981, another tumor in the spinal cord was treated with radiation. The ensuing remission was temporary, and the patient died with disseminated DUNHL on January 15, 1982.

Patient 2: A 33-year-old nurse developed a tumor in his left lower jaw in October 1981. Penicillin was given for a suspected abscess, but the mass enlarged. A biopsy on November 24 disclosed DUNHL. Tumor cells contained surface IgM, kappa type, indicating a B-cell

65

tumor. The tumor involved a left axillary lymph node, the retroperitoneum, the bone marrow, and the meninges. Generalized "reactive" lymphadenopathy and mild spenomegaly were present. Systemic and intratecal chemotherapy led to temporary tumor regression; the patient relapsed and died in March 1982.

Patient 3: A 35-year-old janitor developed an enlarged cervical lymph node in October 1981. A dental extraction was performed for a suspected abscess, but lymphadenopathy persisted. A biopsy on December 12 revealed DUNHL. Tumor cells contained surface IgM, kappa type. Tumor was detected in the mediastinum, retroperitoneum, both kidneys, bone marrow, and meninges. Moderate generalized lymphadenopathy and splenomegaly were present. Systemic and intrathecal chemotherapy led to rapid tumor regression; however, this patient has recently relapsed.

Patient 4: A 24-year-old clerk developed backache and fatigue in November 1981. On January 21, 1982, an exploratory laparotomy showed DUNHL with extensive retroperitoneal involvement. Tumor cells contained surface IgM, kappa type. Combination chemotherapy has led to complete remission.

All these patients were homosexual males living in San Francisco. They had no known contact with each other, had no known sexual partners in common, and had no known contact with patients with Kaposi's sarcoma (KS). Each gave a history of a lifestyle that included use of such drugs as nitrite inhalants, amphetamines, and marijuana. Medical histories indicated that all 4 patients had had 1 or more of such infections as hepatitis B, anal warts, gonorrhea, and syphilis. All patients had generalized lymphadenopathy, and 3 had spenomegaly of uncertain duration. Detailed virology and immunology studies are in progress.

Reported by JL Ziegler, MD, G Wagner, MD, VA Medical Center, San Francisco, JS Greenspan, BDS, PhD, MRC Path, EJ Shillitoe, BDS, PhD, D Greenspan, BDS, J Beckstead, MD, C Cassavant, PhD, D Abrams, MD, W Chan, DDS, S Silverman, DDS, F Lozada, DDS, University of California San Francisco, School of Medicine and Dentistry, L Drew, MD, E Rosenbaum, MD, R Miner, BS, L Mintz, MD, J Gershow, MD, R Weiss, MD, Mt. Zion Hospital, San Francisco, K Yamamoto, MD, K Chich, MD, St. Mary's Hospital San Francisco, S Dritz, MD, MPH, Dept of Public Health, San Francisco, D Austin, MD, MPH, Dept of Health Svcs, Berkeley, J Chin, MD, State Epidemiologist, California Dept of Health Svcs; W McGuire, MD, University of Illinois Hospital, I Iossifides, MD, Abraham Lincoln School of Medicine, Chicago, BJ Francis, MD, State Epidemiologist, Illinois State Dept of Public Health; J Costa, MD, National Cancer Institute, National Institutes of Health; Chronic Disease Div, Center for Environmental Health, Center for Infectious Diseases, the Task Force on Kaposi's Sarcoma and Opportunistic Infections, CDC.

Editorial Note: Since July 1981, CDC has received reports of 162 cases of Kaposi's sarcoma among young homosexual males; the above report documents the possible appearance of a second unusual malignancy among this group of young males — i.e., DUNHL, a B-cell lymphoma(3).

The difficulty in distinguishing DUNHL histologically from Burkitt's lymphoma (BL)(3), a tumor often associated with Epstein-Barr virus, and the lack of consensus on the classification of non-Hodgkin's lymphoma (NHL)(4) make the precise determination of incidence difficult. About 0.7%-2.4% of all cases of NHL are DUNHL(4,5) — for a crude incidence rate of 0.06-0.21/100,000 population/year. No cases of DUNHL and only 1 case of BL were reported in 1977-1980 among 20-39 year olds to the Surveillance Epidemiology and End Results Cancer Registry in the San Francisco-Oakland Standard Metropolitan Statistical Area, emphasizing the unusual occurrence of 4 cases within 10 months in the San Francisco homosexual male population. CDC has also recently received a report from Chicago of another case of DUNHL affecting a young homosexual male.

Underlying immune deficiency appears to be the common denominator for the development of the opportunistic infections and tumors associated with the KSOI syndrome(6-8). A similar syndrome, with an increased risk for NHL but a different time course and spectrum of opportunistic diseases, appears among renal allograft recipients(4,9). Lymphoreticular tumors also occur much more frequently among patients with primary immunodeficiency disorders(4). The cause of the acquired cellular immunodeficiency among homosexual males is being studied.

This report of DUNHL suggests that more than one kind of tumor may occur in association with the KSOI syndrome; assessment of these patients' immunologic findings will help to document the relationship between such tumors and the KSOI syndrome. The full range of potential outcomes (i.e., opportunistic tumors and infections) is probably only now being elucidated. There have also been recent case reports of other malignancies affecting the homosexual population, including carcinoma of the anal rectum(10) and squamous cell carcinoma of the oral cavity(11,12). The excess of carcinoma of the anus and anal rectum appears to antedate the onset of KSOI syndrome(13). The relationship between these malignancies and the KSOI syndrome is uncertain.

Many homosexual males with persistent, unexplained, generalized lymphadenopathy and biopsies reportedly demonstrating only reactive hyperplasia have also been reported to CDC and are under active investigation(14). Homosexual males with clinical findings similar to DUNHL or lymphadenopathic KS(15) should be carefully evaluated and followed.

References
1. Durack DT. Opportunistic infections and Kaposi's sarcoma in homosexual men. N Eng J. Med 1981;305:1465-7. Editorial.
2. Centers for Disease Control Task Force on Kaposi's Sarcoma and Opportunistic Infections. Epidemiologic aspects of the current outbreak of Kaposi's sarcoma and opportunistic infection. N Eng J Med 1982; 306:248-52.
3. Grogan TM, Warnke RA, Kaplan HS. A comparative study of Burkitt's and non-Burkitt's "undifferentiated" malignant lymphoma. Cancer 1982;49:1817-28.
4. Greene MH. Non-Hodgkin's lymphoma and mycosis fungoides. In: Cancer Epidemiology and Prevention. M Schottenfeld, JF Fraumeni, eds, WB Saunders, Philadelphia 1982:754-78.
5. National Cancer Institute. Surveillance epidemiology and results. Incidence and mortality data 1973-1977. Monograph 57. U. S.

Department of Health and Human Resources. NIH Publication No. 81-2330. National Cancer Institute. Bethesda, Maryland 20205. 1981.

6. *Gottlieb MS, Schroff R, Schauker HM, et al. Pneumocystis carinii pneumonia and mucosal candidiasis in previously healthy homosexual men: evidence of a new acquired cellular immunodeficiency. N Eng J Med 1981;305:1425-31.*

7. *Masur H, Michelis MA, Greene, JB, et al. An outbreak of community-acquired Pneumocystis carinii pneumonia: initial manifestations of cellular immune dysfunction. N Eng J Med 1981;305:1431-8.*

8. *Siegal FP, Lopez C, Hammer GS, et al. Severe acquired immunodeficiency in male homosexuals, manifested by chronic perianal ulcerative Herpes simplex lesions. N Eng J Med 1981;305:1439-44.*

9. *Penn I. Malignant lymphomas in organ transplant recipients. Transplant Proc 1981;13:736-8.*

10. *Leach RD, Ellis H. Carcinoma of the rectum in male homosexuals. J R Soc Med 1981; 74-490-1.*

11. *Conant MA, Volberding P, Fletcher V, Lozada Fl, Silverman S. Squamous cell carcinoma in sexual partner of Kaposi sarcoma patient. Lancet 1982;1:286. Letter.*

12. *Lozada F, Silverman S, Conant MA. New outbreak of oral tumors, malignancies and infectious diseases strikes young male homosexuals. Journal of California Dental Association 1982;10:39-42.*

13. *Daling, JR, Weiss NS, Klopfenstein LL, Cochran LE, Chow WH, Daifuku R. Correlates of homosexual behavior and the incidence of anal cancer. JAMA 1982;247:1988-90.*

14. *CDC. Persistent, generalized lymphadenopathy among homosexual males. MMWR 1982;31:249-51.*

15. *Scully RE, Marck EJ, McNeely BU. Case records of the Massachusetts General Hospital. N Eng J Med 1982;306:657-68.*

June 11, 1982

Update on Kaposi's Sarcoma and Opportunistic Infections in Previously Healthy Persons
— United States

Between June 1, 1981, and May 28, 1982, CDC received reports of 355 cases* of Kaposi's sarcoma (KS) and/or serious opportunistic infections (OI), especially Pneumocystis carinii pneumonia (PCP), occurring in previously healthy persons between 15 and 60 years of age. Of the 355, 381 (79%) were homosexual (or bisexual) men, 41 (12%) were heterosexual men, 20 (6%) were men of unknown sexual orientation, and 13 (4%) were heterosexual women. This proportion of heterosexuals (16%) is higher than previously described(1).

Five states — California, Florida, New Jersey, New York, and Texas — accounted for 86% of the reported cases. The rest were reported by 15 other states. New York was reported as the state of residence for 51% of homosexual male patients, 49% of the heterosexual males, and 46% of the females. The median age at onset of symptoms was 36.0 years for homosexual men, 31.5 years for heterosexual men, and 29.0 years for women. The distribution of homosexual and heterosexual KSOI cases by date of onset is shown in Figure 2. Overall, 69% of all reported cases have had onset after January 1, 1981.

PCP accounted for a significantly higher proportion of the diagnoses for both male (63%) and female (73%) heterosexual patients than for homosexual patients (42%) (p less than 0.05). The ratio of homosexual to heterosexual males with PCP only, by year of onset of symptoms, was 5:1 in 1980, 3:1 in 1981 and 4:1 thus far in 1982. Reported case-fatality ratios for PCP cases with onset in 1980 and 1981 were 85% and 47%, respectively, for homosexual men and 67% and 41% for heterosexual men. The distribution of PCP cases by diagnosis, sexual orientation, race, and overall case-fatality ratio is shown in Table 1.

Both male and female heterosexual PCP patients were more likely than homosexual patients to be black or Hispanic (p=0.0001). Of patients with PCP for whom drug-use information was known, 14% of homosexual men had used intravenous drugs at some time compared with 63% of heterosexual men (p=0.001) and 57% of heterosexual women (p=0.001)(Table1).

Reported by Task Force on Kaposi's Sarcoma and Opportunistic Infections, Field Svcs. Div, Epidemiology Program Office, CDC.

Editorial Note: Sexual orientation information was obtained from patients by their physicians, and the accuracy of reporting cannot be determined; therefore, comparisons between KSOI cases made on the basis of sexual orientation must be interpreted cautiously. Similarities between homosexual and heterosexual cases in diagnoses and geographic and temporal distribution suggest that all are part of the same epidemic. Masur et al(2) also reported that lymphocyte dysfunction and lymphopenia were similar in heterosexual and homosexual cases of PCP. However, differences in race, proportion of PCP cases, and intravenous drug use suggest that risk factors may be different for these groups. A laboratory and interview study of heterosexual patients with diagnosed KS, PCP, or other OI is in progress to determine whether their cellular immune function, results of virologic studies, medical history, sexual practices, drug use, and lifestyle are similar to those of homosexual patients.

References

1. *CDC. Follow-up on Kaposi's sarcoma and Pneumocystis pneumonia. MMWR 1981;30:409-10.*

2. *Masur H, Michelis M, Greene JB, et al. An outbreak of community-acquired Pneumocystis carinii pneumonia: initial manifestations of*

---

*A case is defined as illness in a person who 1) has either biopsy-proven KS or biopsy- or culture-proven, life-threatening opportunistic infection, 2) is under age 60, and 3) has no history of either immunosuppressive underlying illness or immunosuppressive therapy.

cellular immune dysfunction. N Engl J Med 1981; 305:1431-8.

FIGURE 2. Cases of KSOI by specific diagnosis, year of onset, sex, and sexual orientation, United States, 1978-1982

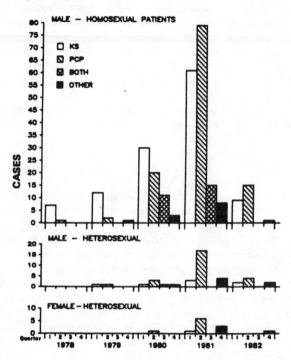

*A case is defined as illness in a person who 1) has either biopsy-proven KS or biopsy- or culture-proven, life-threatening opportunistic infection, 2) is under age 60, and 3) has no history of either immunosuppressive underlying illness or immunosuppressive therapy.

TABLE 1. Reported cases of Pneumocystis carinii pneumonia in previously healthy persons, June 1, 1981-May 28, 1982, United States

		Race				
	Total	White	Black	Hispanic	Case-fatality ratio	IV-Drug Use**
Homosexual men*	118	80	22	15	51%	11/80 (14%)
Heterosexual men*	26	8	11	6	35%	17/26 (65%)
Heterosexual women*	8	1	4	2	50%	4/7 (57%)

*Race data lacking for 1 case

**Data not available on all cases

June 18, 1982

A Cluster of Kaposi's Sarcoma and Pneumocystis carinii Pneumonia among Homosexual Males Residents
Los Angeles and Orange Counties, California

In the period June 1, 1981-April 12, 1982, CDC received reports of 19 cases of biopsy-confirmed Kaposi's sarcoma (KS) and/or Pneumocystis carinii pneumonia (PCP) among previously healthy homosexual male residents of Los Angeles and Orange Counties, California. Following an unconfirmed report of possible associations among cases in southern California, interviews were conducted with all 8 of the patients still living and with the close friends of 7 of the other 11 patients who had died.

Data on sexual partners were obtained for 13 patients, 8 with KS and 5 with PCP. For any patient to be considered as a sexual contact of another person, the reported exposures of that patient had to be either substantiated or not denied by the other person involved in the relationship (or by a close friend of that person).

Within 5 years of the onset of symptoms, 9 patients (6 with KS and 3 with PCP) had had sexual contact with other patients with KS or PCP. Seven patients from Los Angeles County had had sexual contact with other patients from Los Angeles County, and 2 from Orange County had had sexual contact with 1 patient who was not a resident of California. Four of the 9 patients had been exposed to more than 1 patient who had KS or PCP. Three of the 6 patients with KS developed their symptoms after sexual contact with persons who already had symptoms of KS. One of these patients developed symptoms of KS 9 months after sexual contact, another patient developed symptoms 13 months after contact, and a third patient developed symptoms 22 months after contact.

The other 4 patients in the group of 13 had no known sexual contact with reported cases. However, 1 patient with KS had an apparently healthy sexual partner in common with 2 persons with PCP; 1 patient with KS reported having had sexual contact with 2 friends of the non-Californian with KS; and 2 patients with PCP had most of their anonymous contacts (greater than or equal to 80%) with persons in bathhouses attended frequently by other persons in Los Angeles with KS or PCP.

The 9 patients from Los Angeles and Orange counties directly linked to other patients are part of an interconnected series of cases that may include 15 additional patients (11 with KS and 4 with PCP) from 8 other cities. The non-Californian with KS mentioned earlier is part of this series. In addition to having had sexual contact with 2 patients with KS from Orange County, this patient said he had sexual contact with 1 patient with KS and 1 patient with PCP from New York City and 2 of the 3 patients with PCP from Los Angeles County.

Reported by S Fannin, MD, County of Los Angeles Dept of Health Svcs, MS Gottlieb, MD, UCLA School of Medicine, JD Weisman, DO, E Rogolsky, MD, Los Angeles, T Prendergast, MD, County of Orange Dept of Public Health and Medical Svcs, J Chin, MD, State Epidemiologist, California Dept of Health Svcs; AE Friedman-Kien, MD, L Laubenstein, MD, New York University Medical Center, S Friedman, MD, New York City Dept of Health, R Rothenberg, MD, State Epidemiologist, New York Health Dept; Task Force on Kaposi's Sarcoma and Opportunistic Infections, CDC.

Editorial Note: An estimated 185,000-415,000 homosexual males live in Los Angeles County.* Assuming that they had a median of 13.5 to 50 different sexual partners per year over the past 5 years,** the probability that 7 of 11 patients with KS or PCP would have sexual contact with any one of the other 16 reported patients in Los Angeles County would seem to be remote. The probability that 2 patients with KS living in different parts of Orange County would have sexual contact with the same non-Californian with KS would appear to be even lower. Thus, observations in Los Angeles and Orange counties imply the existence of an unexpected cluster of cases.

The cluster in Los Angeles and Orange counties was identified on the basis of sexual contact. One hypothesis consistent with the observations reported here is that infectious agents are being sexually transmitted among homosexually active males. Infectious agents not yet identified may cause the acquired cellular immunodeficiency that appears to underlie KS and/or PCP among homosexual meals(3-6). If infectious agents cause these illnesses, sexual partners of patients may be at increased risk of developing KS and/or PCP.

Another hypothesis to be considered is that sexual contact with patients with KS or PCP does not lead directly to acquired cellular immunodeficiency, but simply indicates a certain style of life. The number of homosexually active males who share this lifestyle may be much smaller than the number of homosexual males in the general population.

Exposure to some substance (rather than an infectious agent) may eventually lead to immunodeficiency among a subset of the homosexual male population that shares a particular style of life. For example, Marmor et al. recently reported that exposure to amyl nitrite was associated with an increased risk of KS in New York City(7). Exposure to inhalant sexual stimulants, central-nervous-system stimulants, and a variety of other "street" drugs was common among males belonging to the cluster of cases of KS and PCP in Los Angeles and Orange counties.

---

*Estimates of the homosexual male population are derived from Kinsey et al.(1) who reported that 8% of adult males are exclusively homosexual and that 18% have at least as much homosexual as heterosexual experience for at least 3 years between the ages of 16 and 55 years; and the U. S. Bureau of the Census, which reported that approximately 2,304,000 males between the ages of 18 and 64 years lived in Los Angeles County in 1980.

**Estimates of sexual activity are derived from data collected by Jay and Young(2), indicating that 130 homosexual male respondents in Los Angeles had a median of 13.5 different sexual partners in 1976, and from CDC data showing that 13 patients with KS and/or PCP in the Los Angeles area tended to report having more sexual partners in the year before onset of symptoms (median=50) than did homosexual males surveyed by Jay and Young.

References

1. Kinsey AC, Pomeroy WB, Martin CE. Sexual behavior in the human male. Philadelphia: WB Saunders, 1948:650-1.
2. Jay K, Young A. The gay report. New York: Summit, 1979.
3. Friedman-Kien AE. Disseminated Kaposi's sarcoma syndrome in young homosexual men. Am Acad Dermatol 1981;5:468-71.
4. Gottlieb MS, Schroff R, Schanker HM, et al. Pneumocystis carinii pneumonia and mucosal candidiasis in previously healthy homosexual men. N Engl J Med 1981;305:1425-31.
5. Masur H, Michelis MA, Greene JB, et al. An outbreak of community-acquired Pneumocystis carinii pneumonia. N Engl J Med 1981; 305:1431-8.
6. Siegal FP, Lopez C, Hammer GS, et al. Severe acquired immunodeficiency in male homosexuals, manifested by chronic perianal ulcerative herpes simplex lesions. N Engl J Med 1981;305:1439-44.
7. Marmor M., Friedman-Kien AE, Laubenstein L, et al. Risk factors for Kaposi's sarcoma in homosexual men. Lancet 1982;1:1083-7.

July 9, 1982

Opportunistic Infections and Kaposi's Sarcoma among Haitians in the United States

Reports of opportunistic infections and Kaposi's sarcoma among Haitians residing in the United States have recently been received at CDC. A total of 34 cases in 5 states have been reported to date.

Florida: From April 1, 1980, through June 20, 1082, 19 Haitian patients admitted to Jackson Memorial Hospital, Miami, had culture, biopsy, or autopsy evidence of opportunistic infections, and 1 other patient had biopsy- and autopsy-confirmed Kaposi's sarcoma. The infections identified included Pneumocystis carinii pneumonia (6 patients), cryptococcal meningitis or fungemia(4), toxoplasmosis of the central nervous system (CNS)(7), Candida albicans esophagitis(7) and thrus(5), esophageal or disseminated cytomegalovirus infection(3), progressive herpes simplex virus infection(1), disseminated tuberculosis(8), and chronic enteric Isospora belli infection(2). Fourteen patients had multiple opportunistic infections. Three patients had recurring infection. The clinical course has been severs; 10 patients have died. The type of infection was initially recognized at autopsy for 6 patients.

The 20 patients ranged in age from 22 to 43 years (mean 28.4 years); 17 were males. All the patients had been born in Haiti and had resided in the Miami-Dade County area for period ranging from 1 month to 7 years (median 20.5 months).

When initially seen, 18 of the 20 patients had peripheral lymphopenia (less than 1,000 lymphocytes/mm^3). Skin tests performed on 17 patients with various combinations of tuberculin, mumps, streptokinase/streptodornase, Candida, and Trichophyton antigens were all negative. Immunologic studies at CDC on specimens from the 11 patients tested showed severe T-cell dysfunction. Monoclonal antibody analysis of peripheral-blood T-cell subsets revealed a marked decrease of the T-helper cell subset with inversion of the normal ratio of T-helper to T-suppressor cells.

Of the 7 patients with histologically confirmed toxoplasmosis of the CNS, 5 have died. Because there was no history of underlying conditions or drugs associated with immunosuppression, CNS toxoplasmosis was not considered in the premortem diagnosis of the first 4 cases. Pathology findings for all these patients were confirmed with an immuno-peroxidase method for toxoplasmosis and, in one instance, with electron microscopy as well. Tachyzoites were the predominant form of the parasite observed; encysted forms were rare or absent in many tissue blocks.

In addition to the 20 cases reported from Miami, A Haitian female from Naples, Floria, was reported to have P. carinii pneumonia.

New York: From July 1, 1981, through May 31, 1982, 10 Haitian residents of Brooklyn were diagnosed as having the following opportunistic infections: P. carinii pneumonia (5 patients), CNS toxoplasmosis(2), disseminated cryptococcosis(1), esophageal candidiasis(1), and disseminated tuberculosis(2). None had any underlying disease or history of therapy known to cause immunosuppression. Five died of their infections.

All 10 patients were males and ranged in age from 22 to 37 years. Eight stated they were heterosexual. the sexual orientation of the other 2 was not known. One patient gave a history of intravenous (IV) drug abuse; 8 denied drug abuse, and for 1, no information was available on drug use. The 10 had resided in the United States for periods ranging from 3 months to 8 years (the majority, for 2 years or less). At least 1 patient had onset of illness before arriving in the United States. Immunologic studies performed at CDC on specimens from 2 patients showed results comparable to those for the 11 patients from Miami.

Other States: Opportunistic infections or Kaposi's sarcoma were also reported for 3 other Haitians located in California, Georgia, and New Jersey. All 3 were heterosexual males who denied IV drug abuse. One patient had P. carinii pneumonia, another had Kaposi's sarcoma, and the third had esophageal candidiasis.

Reported by GT Hensley, MD, LB Moskowitz, MD, AE Pitchenik, MD, MA Fischl, MD, SZ Tabei MD, P Kory, MD, MJ post, MD, FK Conley, MD (Stanford University School of Medicine), G Dickinson, MD, D Becker, MD, A Fournier, MD, M O'Connell, MD, G Scott, MD, University of Miami School of Medicine, RA Morgan, MD, JQ Cleveland, MD, Dade County Health Dept, H Tennis, Metropolitan Dade County, HT Janowski, MPH, RA Gunn, MD, MPH, State Epidemiologist, Florida Dept of Health and Rehabilitative Svcs; J Viera, MD, S Landesman, MD, E Frank, MD, J Nadler, MD, Kings County Hospital, SUNY Downstate Medical Center, Brooklyn, C Metroka, MD, T Nash, MD, New York Hospital, SM Friedman, MD, DJ Sencer, MD, New York City Dept of Health, R Rothenberg, MD, State Epidemiologist, New York State

Dept of Health; T Howard, MD, Cedars-Sinai Medical Center, M Gottlieb, MD, UCLA Medical Center, S Fannin, MD, Los Angeles County Dept of Health Svcs, J Chin, MD, State Epidemiologist, California Dept of Health Svcs; R Kapila, MD, New Jersey College of Medicine and Dentistry, IC Guerrero, WE Parkin, DVM, State Epidemiologist, New Jersey Dept of Health; J Hawkins, MD, Medical College of Georgia, RK Sikes, DVM, State Epidemiologist, Georgia Dept of Human Resources; Div of Parasitic Diseases, Div of Host Factors, Center for Infectious Diseases, Field Svcs Div, Epidemiology Program Office, Task Force on Kaposi's Sarcoma and Opportunistic Infections, CDC.

Editorial Note: The occurrence of severe opportunistic infections among 32 Haitians recently entering the United States is a new phenomenon. The in vitro immunologic findings and the high mortality rate (nearly 50%) for these patients are similar to the pattern recently described among homosexual males and IV Drug Abusers(1-4). None of the 23 Haitian males questioned reported homosexual activity, and only 1 of 26 gave a history of IV drug abuse — substantially lower than the prevalence reported for heterosexual patients of other racial/ethnic groups who had Kaposi's sarcoma or opportunistic infections. Of the 34 patients discussed above with opportunistic infections or Kaposi's sarcoma, 30 (88%) were males. All patients were between 20 and 45 years of age. Data from medical screening of 10,780 Haitians entering the United States between March and November 1980 indicated that 73% were adult males. Only 2% of those screened were less than 12 years old, and over 90% were less than 45 years old(5).

The occurrence of opportunistic infections among adult Haitians with no history of underlying immunosuppressive therapy or disease has not been reported previously. However, 11 cases of disseminated Kaposi's sarcoma have been diagnosed by dermatologists in Port au Prince, Haiti, over a period of 2½ years(6). The reason for the high prevalence of disseminated tuberculosis among the group of patients discussed above is not know; but a high prevalence of tuberculosis has been documented among recent Haitian entrants(7), and the disease has been reported to disseminate more frequently among persons who are immunocomprised(8,9).

To date, it has not been established whether the cases of toxoplasmosis represent reactivation of old lesions acquired in Haiti or whether they are progressive primary infections acquired in the United States. However, serum specimens obtained from 2 patients in Miami and tested at CDC by indirect immuno-fluorescence (IIF) were negative for IgM antibody to Toxoplasma. This suggests that the infections of these 2 patients were not recently acquired. Serologic tests such as the IIF may be helpful in establishing or excluding a diagnosis of toxoplasmosis for patients with CNS symptoms. Tachyzoites in tissue specimens can be visualized more effectively using Giemsa stain or a recently developed immuno-peroxidase methos(10) than with the standard hemotoxylin and erosin staining.

It is not clear whether this outbreak is related to similar outbreaks among homosexual males, IV drug abusers, and others, but the clinical and immunologic pictures appear quite similar. CDC is currently collaborating with local investigators to define this problem and identify risk factors.

Physicians who care for Haitian patients should be aware that opportunistic infections may occur in this population. Health-care providers who diagnose opportunistic infectios or Kaposi's sarcoma among persons who do not have underlying disease and are not on immunosuppressive therapy are requested to report such cases to CDC through their appropriate state and local health departments.

References

1. CDC. Follow-up on Kaposi's sarcoma and pneumocystis pneumonia. MMWR 1981;30:409-10.
2. CDC. Update on Kaposi's sarcoma and opportunistic infections in previously healthy persons — United States. MMWR 1982;31: 294,300-1.
3. Masur H. Michelis MA, Greene JB, et al. An outbreak of community-acquired Pneumocystis carinii pneumonia: initial manifestation of cellular immune dysfunction. N Engl J Med 1981; 305:1431-8.
4. Gottlief MS, Schroff R, Schanker HM, et al. Pneumocystis carinii pneumonia and mucosal candidiasis in previously healthy homosexual men: evidence of a new acquired cellular immunodeficiency. N Engl J Med 1981;305:1425-31.
5. U. S. Public Health Service. Report on the medical status of Haitian entrants processed at the Federal Processing Center, FCI, Miami. March 7, 1980 to November 10, 1980. Unpublished report, 1980.
6. Liautaud B, Laroche C, Duvivier J, Pean-Guichard C. Le sarcome de Kaposi (maladie de Kaposi) est-il frequent en Haiti? Presented at the 18th Congres des Medecins francophones de l'hemisphere americain: Port au Prince, Haiti, April 1982.
7. Pitchenik AE, Russell BW, Cleary T, et al. The prevalence of tuberculosis and drug resistance among Haitians. New Engl J Med (in press).
8. Kaplan MH, Armstrong D, Rosen P. Tuberculosis complicating neoplastic disease: a review of 201 cases. Cancer 1974;33:850-8.
9. Williams DM, Krick, JA, Remington JS. Pulmonary infection in the compromised host: part II. Am Rev Resp Dis 1976; 114:593-627.
10. Conley FK, Jenkins KA, Remington JS. Toxoplasma gondii infection of the central nervous system; use of the peroxidase-antiperoxidase method to demostrate toxoplasma in formalin fixed, parafin embedded tissue sections. Human Pathol 1981;12:690-8.

July 16, 1982

Pneumocystis carinii Pneumonia among Persons with Hemophilia A

CDC recently received reports of three cases of Pneumocystis carinii pneumonia among patients with hemophilia A and without other underlying disease. Two have died; one remains critically ill. All three were heterosexual males; none had a history of intravenous (IV) drug abuse. All had lymphopenia, and the two patients who were specifically tested have had in vitro laboratory evidence of cellular immune deficiency. The case reports follow.

Patient 1: A 62-year-old resident of Westchester County, New York, with a history of chronic hepatitis had received frequent injections of Factor VIII concentrate for severe hemophilia for many years. In February 1981, he began to experience weight loss and vague right upper quadrant abdominal discomfort associated with laboratory evidence of increasing hepatic dysfunction. In December 1981, while hospitalized in Miami, Florida, for elective knee surgery, he complained of cough and fever. He was lymphopenic, and chest X-ray revealed interstitial infiltrates compatible with viral pneumonia. He was discharged in late December after a brief course of corticosteroids associated with overall clinical improvement. He returned in severe respiratory distress a few days later. Open lung biopsy on January 5 revealed P. carinii, for which he received sulfamethoxazole/trimethoprim (SMZ/TMP) during the 2 weeks before death. P. carinii pneumonia and micronodular cirrhosis were documented at post-mortem examination.

Patient 2: A 59-year-old lifelong resident of Denver, Colorado, noted the onset of gradual weight loss, dysphagia associated with pharyngitis, aphthous-like ulcers, and anterior cervical adenopathy begining in October 1980. As a patient with severe hemophilia, he had received frequent injections of Factor VIII concentrate for several years. Weight loss continued over a period of months. Oropharyngeal candidiasis was diagnosed in February 1982. He was hospitalized in May 1982 with symptoms including nausea, vomiting, and recurrent fever. Pneumonia was diagnosed and P. carinii and cytomegalovirus (CMV) were repeatedly identified from lung tissue or bronchial secretions using histopathologic and culture techniques. Therapy with SMZ/TMP and pentamidine isethionate continued until death on July 5, 1982. Laboratory evidence for cellular immune dysfunction included absent mitogen responses and depletion of the T-helper lymphocyte cell population, relative increase in T-suppressor cells, and resultant inverted T-helper/T-suppressor ratio.

Patient 3: A previously healthy 27-year-old lifelong resident of northeastern Ohio developed fever, urinary frequency and urgency, and extreme lassitude in July 1981. He had frequently received parenteral Factor VIII concentrate for severe hemophilia. Bilateral pneumonia was diagnosed in October 1981, and open lung biopsy revealed P. carinii. He responded successfully to a 3-week course of SMZ/TMP. In February 1982, he received ketoconazole to suppress repeated episodes of oral candidiasis. He was hospitalized again in April with fever, splenomegaly, anemia, and lymphopenia. An extensive tumor work-up (including laparotomy) did not uncover an underlying malignancy. Cultures of bone marrow, liver, mesenteric lymph nodes, and blood grew Mycobacterium avium. In vitro immunological testing in March indicated a reduction in absolute number of circulating T-cells. Subsequent, more extensive testing documented the lack of lymphocyte responsiveness to mitogens, absolute and relative decrease in T-helper cells, relative increase in T-suppressor cells, and resultant inverted T-helper/T-suppressor ratio.

For each patient, records of the administration of Factor VIII concentrate were reviewed to determine manufacturer and lot numbers. No two of the patients are known to have received concentrate from the same lots.

Reported by: NJ Ehrenkranz, MD, South Florida Hospital Consortium for Infection Control, J Rubini, MD, Cedars of Lebanon Hospital, Miami, R Gunn, MD, State Epidemiologist, Florida Dept of Health and Rehabilitative Svcs; CR Horsburgh, MD, T Collins, MD, U Hasiba, MD, W Hathaway, MD, University of Colorado School of Medicine, W Doig, MD, R Hopkins, MD, State Epidemiologist, Colorado Dept of Health; J Elliott, MD, W Hoppes, MD, I Patel, MD, Aultman Hospital, Canton, CE Krill, MD, Children's Hospital, Akron, T Halpin, MD, State Epidemiologist, Ohio Dept of Health; Field Services Div, Epidemiology Program Office, Div of Host Factors, Center for Infectious Diseases, Task Force on Kaposi's Sarcoma and Opportunistic Infections, CDC.

Editorial Note: Pneumocystis carinii pneumonia has not been previously reported among hemophilia patients who have had no other underlying diseases and have not had therapy commonly associated with immunosuppression. A review of the Parasitic Disease Drug Service s records of request for pentamidine isethionate for 1980-1982 failed to identify hemophilia among the underlying disorders of patients for whom pentamidine was requested for Pneumocystis carinii therapy.

The clinical and immunologic features these three patients share are strikingly similar to those recently observed among certain individuals from the following groups: homosexual males, heterosexuals who abuse IV drugs, and Haitians who recently entered the United States.(1-3) Although the cuase of the severe immune dysfunction is unknown, the occurrence among the three hemophiliac cases suggests the possible transmission of an agent through blood products.

Hemophilia A is a sex-linked, inherited disorder characterized by a deficiency in Factor VIII activity. There are an estimated 20,000 patients with hemophilia A in the United States(4). Severity of disease is classified according to percentage of endogenous Factor VIII activity. Approximately 60% of the 20,000 are classified as severe, and 40% are classified as moderate(4). Factor VIII deficiency can be treated with intravenous administration of exogenous Factor VIII as either cryoprecipate made from individual units of fresh frozen plasma or lyophilized Factor VIII concentrate manufactured from plasma pools collected from as many as a thousand or more donors.

CDC has notified directors of hemophilia centers about these cases and, with the National Hemophilia Foundation, has initiated collaborative surveillance. A Public Health Service advisory committee is being formed to consider the implication of these findings. Physicians diagnosing opportunistic infections in hemophilia patients who have not received antecedent immunosuppressive therapy are encouraged to report them to the CDC through local and state health departments.

References
1.   CDC. Follow-up on Kaposi's sarcoma and Pneumocystis pneumonia. MMWR 1981;30:409-10.
2.   CDC. Update on Kaposi's sarcoma and opportunistic infections in previously healthy persons — United States. MMWR 1982;31: 294,300-1.
3.   CDC. Opportunistic infections and Kaposi's sarcoma among Haitians in the United States. MMWR 1982;31:353-4,360-1.
4.   Petit CR, Klein HG. Hemophilia, hemophiliacs and the health care delivery system. National Heart and Lung Institute, Division of

Blood Diseases and Resources, Office of Prevention, Control, and Education. DHEW Publication No. (NIH) 76-871, 1976.

September 24, 1982

Update on Acquired Immune Deficiency Syndrome (AIDS) — United States

Between June 1, 1981, and September 15, 1982, CDC received reports of 593 cases of acquired immune deficiency syndrome (AIDS).* Death occurred in 243 cases (41%).

Analysis of reported AIDS cases shows tht 51% had Pneumocystis carinii pneumonia (PCP) without Kaposi's sarcoma (KS)(with or without other "opportunistic" infections [OOI]; and 12% has OOI with neither PCP nor KS. The overall mortality rate for cases of PCP without KS (47%) was more than twice that for cases of KS without PCP (21%), while the rate for cases of both PCP and KS (68%) was more than three times as great. The mortality rate for OOI with neither KS nor PCP was 48%.

The incidence of AIDS by date of diagnosis (assuming an almost constant population at risk) has roughly doubled every half-year since the second half of 1979 (Table 1). An average of one to two cases are now diagnosed every day. Although the overall case-mortality rate for the current total of 593 is 41%, the rate exceeds 60% for cases diagnosed over a year ago.

Almost 80% of reported AIDS cases in the United States were concentrated in six metropolitan areas, predominantly on the east and west coasts of the country (Table 2). This distribution was not simply a reflection of population size in those areas; for example, the number of cases per million population reported from June 1, 1981, to September 15, 1982, in New York City and San Francisco was roughly 10 times greater than that of the entire country. The 593 cases were reported among residents of 27 states and the District of Columbia, and CDC has received additional reports of 41 cases from 10 foreign countries.

Approximately 75% of AIDS cases occurred among homosexual or bisexual males (Table 3), among whom the reported prevalence of intravenous drug abuse was 12%. Among the 20% of known heterosexual cases (males and females), the prevalence of intravenous drug abuse was about 60%. Haitians residing in the United States constituted 6.1% of all cases(2), and 50% of the cases in which both homosexual activity and intravenous drug abuse were denied. Among the 14 AIDS cases involving males under 60 years old who were not homosexuals, intravenous drug abusers, or Haitians, two (14%) had hemophilia A.**(3)

Reported AIDS cases may be separated into groups based on these risk factors: homosexual or bisexual males — 75%, intravenous drug abusers with no history of male homosexual activity — 13%, Haitians with neither a history of homosexuality nor a history of intravenous drug abuse — 6%, persons with hemophilia A who were not Haitians, homosexuals, or intravenous drug abusers — 0.3%, and persons in none of the other groups — 5%.

Reported by the Task Force on Acquired Immune Deficiency Syndrome, CDC.

Editorial Note: CDC defines a case of AIDS as a disease, at least moderately predictive of a defect in cell-mediated immunity, occurring in a persons with no known cause for diminished resistance to that disease. Such diseases include KS, PCP, and serious OOI.*** Diagnoses are considered to fit the case definition only if based on sufficiently reliable methods (generally histology or culture). However, this case definition may not include the full spectrum of AIDS manifestations, which may range from absence of symptoms (despite laboratory evidence of immune deficiency) to non-specific symptoms (e.g., fever, weight loss, generalized, persistent lymphadenopathy)(4) to specific diseases that are insufficiently predictive of cellular immunodeficiency to be included in incidence monitoring (e.g., tuberculosis, oral candidiasis, herpes zoster) to malignant neoplasms that cause, as well as result from, immunodeficiency****(5). Conversely, some patients who are considered AIDS cases on the basis of diseases only moderately predictive of cellular immunodeficiency may not actually be immunodeficient and may not be part of the current epidemic. Absence of a reliable, inexpensive, widely available test for AIDS, however, may make the working case definition the best currently available for incidence monitoring.

Two points in this update deserve emphasis. First, the eventual case-mortality rate of AIDS, a few years after diagnosis, may be far greater than the 41% overall case-mortality rate noted above. Second, the reported incidence of AIDS has continued to increase rapidly. Only a small percentage of cases have none of the identified risk factors (male homosexuality, intravenous drug abuse, Haitian origin, and perhaps hemophilia A). To avoid a reporting bias, physicians should report cases regardless of the absence of these factors.

Physicians aware of patients fitting the case definition for AIDS are requested to report such cases to CDC through their local or state health departments.

---

*Formerly referred to as Kaposi's sarcoma and opportunistic infections in previously healthy persons.(1)

**A third hemophilia with pneumocystosis exceeded the 60-year age limit of the AIDS case definition.

***These infections include pneumonia, meningitis, or encephalitis due to one or more of the following: aspergillosis, candidiasis, cryptococcosis, cytomegalovirus, nocardiosis, strongyloidosis, toxoplasmosis, zygomycosis, or atypical mycobacteriosis (species other than tuberculosis or lepra); esophagitis due to candidiasis, cytomegalovirus, or herpes simplex virus; progressive multifocal leukoencephalopathy; chronic enterocolitis (more than 4 weeks) due to cryptosporidiosis; or unusually extensive mucocutaneous herpes simplex of more than 5 weeks duration.

****CDC encourages reports of any cancer among persons with AIDS and of selected rare lymphomas (Burkitt's or difuse, undifferentiated non-Hodgkins lymphoma) among persons with a risk factor for AIDS. This differs from the request for reports of AIDS cases regardless of the absence of risk factors.

TABLE 1. Reported cases and case-mortality rates of AIDS, by half-year of diagnosis*, 1979-1982, (as of September 15, 1982) -- United States

Half-year of diagnosis		Cases	Deaths	Case-mortality rate (%)
1979	1st half	1	1	100
	2nd half	6	5	83
1980	1st half	17	13	76
	2nd half	26	22	85
1981	1st half	66	46	70
	2nd half	141	79	56
1982	1st half	249	67	27

*Excluding 4 cases with unknown dates of diagnosis

TABLE 2. AIDS cases per million population*, by standard metropolitan statistical area (SMSA) of residence, reported from June 1, 1981 to September 15, 1982 -- United States

SMSA of residence	Cases	Percentage of total	Cases per million population
New York, New York	288	48.6	31.6
San Francisco, California	78	13.2	24.0
Miami, Florida	31	5.2	19.1
Newark, New Jersey	15	2.5	7.6
Houston, Texas	15	2.5	5.2
Los Angeles, California	37	6.2	4.9
Elsewhere (irrespective of SMSA)	129	21.8	0.6
Total	593	100.0	2.6

*From the 1980 Census

TABLE 3. Cases of AIDS, by sexual orientation and intravenous drug abuse, reported from June 1, 1981 to September 15, 1982 -- United States

Sex	Sexual orientation	Cases	Percentage distribution by sexual orientation	Intravenous drug abuse*			Percentage using IV drugs**
				Yes	No	Unknown	
Male	Homosexual or bisexual	445	75.0	42	300	103	12.3
	Heterosexual	84	14.2	49	33	2	59.8
	Unknown	30	5.1	11	11	8	50.0
Female	Heterosexual	34	5.7	20	12	2	62.5
Total		593	100.0	122	356	115	25.5

*Regardless of when the last such activity occurred
**Excluding cases with unknown history of IV drug abuse

References

1. CDC. Update on Kaposi's sarcoma and opportunistic infections in previously healthy persons -- United States. MMWR 1982;31: 294,300-1.
2. CDC. Opportunistic infections and Kaposi's sarcoma among Haitians in the United States. MMWR 1982;31:353-4, 360-1.
3. CDC. Pneumocystis carinii pneumonia among persons with hemophilia A. MMWR 1982;31:365-7.
4. CDC. Persistent, generalized lymphadenopathy among homosexual males. MMWR 1982; 31:249-51.
5. CDC. Diffuse, undifferentiated non-Hodgkins lymphoma among homosexual males -- United States MMWR 1982;31:277-9

Acquired Immune Deficiency Syndrome (AIDS): Precautions for Clinical
and Laboratory Staffs

The etiology of the underlying immune deficiencies seen in AIDS cases is unknown. One hypothesis consistent with current observations is that a transmissible agent may be involved. If so, transmission of the agent would appear most commonly to require intimate, direct contact involving mucosal surfaces, such as sexual contact among homosexual males, or through parenteral spread, such as occurs among intravenous drug abusers and possibly hemophilia patients using Factor VIII products. Airborne spread and interpersonal spread through casual contact do not seem likely. These patterns resemble the distribution of disease and modes of spread of hepatitis B virus, and hepatitis B virus infections occur very frequently among AIDS cases.

There is presently no evidence of AIDS transmission to hospital personnel from contact with affected patients or clinical specimens. Because of concern about a possible transmissible agent, however, interim suggestions are appropriate to guide patient-care and laboratory personnel, including those whose work involves experimental animals. At present, it appears prudent for hospital personnel to use the same precautions when caring for patients with AIDS as those used for patients with hepatitis B virus infection, in which blood and body fluids likely to have been contaminated with blood are considered infective. Specifically, patient-care and laboratory personnel should take precautions to avoid direct contact of skin and mucous membranes with blood, blood products, excretions, secretions, and tissues of persons judged likely to have AIDS. The following precautions do not specifically address out-patient care, dental care, surgery, necropsy, or hemodialysis of AIDS patients. In general, procedures appropriate for patients known to be infected with hepatitis B virus are advised, and blood and organs of AIDS patients should not be donated.

The precautions that follow are advised for persons and specimens from persons with: opportunistic infections that are not associated with underlying immunosuppressive disease or therapy; Kaposi's sarcoma (patients under 60 years of age); chronic generalized lymphadenopathy, unexplained weight loss and/or prolonged unexplained fever in persons who belong to groups with apparently increased risks of AIDS (homosexual males, intravenous drug abusers, Haitian entrants, hemophiliacs); and possible AIDS (hospitalized for evaluation). Hospitals and laboratories should adapt the following suggested precautions to their individual circumstances; these recommendations are not meant to restrict hospitals from implementing additional precautions.

A. **The following precautions are advised in providing care to AIDS patients:**
1. Extraordinary care must be taken to avoid accidental wounds from sharp instruments contaminated with potentially infectious material and to avoid contact of open skin lesions with material from AIDS patients.
2. Gloves should be worn when handling blood specimens, blood-soiled items, body fluids, excretions, and secretions, as well as surfaces, materials, and objects exposed to them.
3. Gowns should be worn when clothing may be soiled with body fluids, blood, secretions, or excretions.
4. Hands should be washed after removing gowns and gloves and before leaving the rooms of known or suspected AIDS patients. Hands should also be washed thoroughly and immediately if they become contaminated with blood.
5. Blood and other specimens should be labeled prominently with a special warning, such as "Blood Precautions" or "AIDS Precautions." If the outside of the specimen container is visibly contaminated with blood, it should be cleaned with a disinfectant (such as a 1:10 dilution of 5.25% sodium hypochlorite [household bleach] with water). All blood specimens should be placed in a second container, such as an impervious bag, for transport. The container or bag should be examined carefully for leaks or cracks.
6. Blood spills should be cleaned up promptly with a disinfectant solution, such as sodium hypochlorite (see above).
7. Articles soiled with blood should be placed in an impervious bag prominently labeled "AIDS Precautions" or "Blood Precautions" before being sent for reprocessing or disposal. Alternatively, such contaminated items may be placed in plastic bags of a particular color designated solely for disposal of infectious westes by the hospital. Disposable items should be incinerated or disposed of in accord with the hospital's policies for disposal of infectious wastes. Reusable items should be reprocessed in accord with hospital policies for hepatitis B virus-contaminated items. Lensed instruments should be sterilized after use on AIDS patients.
8. Needles should not be bent after use, but should be promptly placed in a puncture-resistant container used solely for such disposal. Needles should not be reinserted into their original sheaths before being discarded into the container, since this is a common cause of needle injury.
9. Disposable syringes and needles are preferred. Only needle-locking syringes or one-piece needle-syringe units should be used to aspirate fluids from patients, so that collected fluid can be safely discharged through the needle, if desired. If reusable syringes are employed, they should be decontaminated before reporcessing.
10. A private room is indicated for patients who are too ill to use good hygiene, such as those with profuse diarrhea, fecal incontinence, or altered behavior secondary to central nervous system infections.
    Precautions appropriate for particular infections that concurrently occur in AIDS patients should be added to the above, if needed.
B. **The following precautions are advised for persons performing laboratory tests or studies on clinical specimens or other potentially infectious materials (such as inoculated tissue cultures, embryonated eggs, animal tissues, etc.) from known or suspected AIDS cases:**
1. Mechanical pipetting devices should be used for the manipulation of all liquids in the laboratory. Mouth pipetting should not be allowed.
2. Needles and syringes should be handled as stipulated in Section A(above).

75

3. Laboratory coats, gowns, or uniforms should be worn while working with potentially infectious materials and should be discarded appropriately before leaving the laboratory.

4. Gloves should be worn to avoid skin contact with blood, specimens containing blood, blood-soiled items, body fluids, excretions, and secretions, as well as surfaces, materials, and objects exposed to them.

5. All procedures and manipulations of potentially infectious material should be performed carefully to minimize the creation of droplets and aerosols.

6. Biological safety cabinets (Class I or II) and other primary containment devices (e.g., centrifuge safety cups) are advised whenever procedures are conducted that have a high potential for creating aerosols or infectious droplets. These include centrifuging, blending, sonicating, vigorous mixing, and harvesting infected tissues from animals or embryonated eggs. Fluorescent activated cell sorters generate droplets that could potentially result in infectious aerosols. Translucent plastic shielding between the droplet-collecting area and the equipment operator should be used to reduce the presently uncertain magnitude of this risk. Primary containment devices are also used in handling materials that might contain concentrated infectious agents or organisms in greater quantities than expected in clinical specimens.

7. Laboratory work surfaces should be decontaminated with a disinfectant, such as sodium hypochlorite solution (see A5 above), following any spill of potentially infectious material and at the completion of work activities.

8. All potentially contaminated materials used in laboratory tests should be decontaminated, preferably by autoclaving, before disposal or reprocessing.

9. All personnel should wash their hands following completion of laboratory activities, removal of protective clothing, and before leaving the laboratory.

C. The following additional precautions are advised for studies involving experimental animals inoculated with tissues or other potentially infectious materials from individuals with known or suspected AIDS.

1. Laboratory coats, gowns, or uniforms should be worn by personnel entering rooms housing inoculated animals. Certain nonhuman primates, such as chimpanzees, are prone to throw excreta and to spit at attendants; personnel attending inoculated annimals should wear molded surgical masks and goggles or other equipment sufficient to prevent potentially infective droplets from reaching the mucosal surfaces of their mouths, nares, and eyes. In addition, when handled, other animals may disturb excreta in their bedding. Therefore, the above precautions should be taken when handling them.

2. Personnel should wear gloves for all activities involving direct contact with experimental animals and their bedding and cages. Such manipulations should be performed carefully to minimize the creation of aerosols and droplets.

3. Necropsy of experimental animals sould be conducted by personnel wearing gowns and gloves. If procedures generating aerosols are performed, masks and goggles should be worn.

4. Extraordinary care must be taken to avoid accidental sticks or cuts with sharp instruments contaminated with body fluids or tissues of experimental animals inoculated with material from AIDS patients.

5. Animal cages should be decontaminated, preferably by autoclaving, before they are cleaned and washed.

6. Only needle-locking syringes or one-piece needle-syringe units should be used to inject potentially infectious fluids into experimental animals.

The above precautions are intended to apply to both clinical and research laboratories. Biological safety cabinets and other safety equipment may not be generally available in clinical laboratories. Assistance should be sought from a microbiology laboratory, as needed, to assure containment facilities are adequate to permit laboratory tests to be conducted safely.

Reported by Hospital Infections Program, Div of Viral Diseases, Div of Host Factors, Div of Hepatitis and Viral Enteritis, AIDS Activity, Center for Infectious Diseases, Office of Biosafety, CDC; Div of Safety, National Institutes of Health.

November 12, 1982

Cryptosporidiosis: Assessment of Chemotherapy of Males with Acquired Immune Deficiency Syndrome (AIDS)

Since December 1979, 21 males with severe, protracted diarrhea caused by the parasite, Cryptosporidium, have been reported to CDC by physicians in Boston, Los Angeles, Newark, New York, Philadelphia, and San Francisco, All 21 have acquired immune deficiency syndrome (AIDS); 20 are homosexual; and one is a heterosexual Haitian. Their ages range from 23 to 62 years with a mean of 35.7 years. Most had other opportunistic infections or Kaposi's sarcoma in addition to cryptosporidiosis. Eleven had Pneumocystis carinii pneumonia (PCP); nine had Candida esophagitis; two had a disseminated Mycobacterium avium-intracellulare infection; one had a disseminated cytomegalovirus infection; and two had Kaposi's sarcoma. T-lymphocyte helper-to-suppressor ratios were decreased (less than 0.9) in all 18 patients on whom this test was performed. Fourteen patients have died.

The illness attributed to Cryptosporidium was characterized by chronic, profuse, watery diarrhea. The mean duration of diarrhea was 4 months, often continuing until the patient's death. Bowel movement frequency ranged from six to 25 per day. The estimated maximum volume of stool during illness ranged from 1 to 17 liters per day with a mean of 3.6 liters per day. Diagnosis of cryptosporidiosis was made by histologic examination of small bowel biopsies (13 patients) or large bowel biopsies (four patients), or by stool examination using a sucrose

76

concentration technique (16 patients)(1). More than one type of diagnostic method was positive for several patients.

Table 1 shows the drugs given to the 21 patients while they had diarrhea attributed to Cryptosporidium. Only two patients (9.5%) have had sustained resolution of their diarrhea with negative follow-up stool examinations. The first was being treated with prednisone (60 mg daily) for chronic active hepatitis at the time his diarrhea began. When cryptosporidiosis was diagnosed, he was started on diloxanide furoate (500 mg three times daily for 10 days), and the prednisone was tapered over 2 weeks and then stopped. Two weeks later, his diarrhea was improving; in another 2 weeks, his diarrhea had completely resolved. He has had no diarrhea for 8 months. Follow-up stool examinations 2 weeks and 6 weeks after discontiuation of diloxanide furoate were negative for Cryptosporidium.

TABLE 1. Drugs used to treat males with cryptosporidiosis and AIDS

Drug*	Dose and route of administration[†]	Number of patients	Unchanged n	(%)	Improved[§] n	(%)	Cured[¶] n	(%)
No treatment	—	2	0	(0.0)	2	(100.0)	0	(0.0)
Trimethoprim/ sulfamethoxazole	25 mg/kg QID of sulfamethoxazole	7	7	(100.0)	0	(0.0)	0	(0.0)
Trimethoprim/ sulfamethoxazole	800 mg PO BID of sulfamethoxazole	4	4	(100.0)	0	(0.0)	0	(0.0)
Furazolidone	100 mg PO QID	6	4	(66.7)	1	(16.7)	1	(16.7)
Furazolidone	300 mg PO QID	1	1	(100.0)	0	(0.0)	0	(0.0)
Metronidazole	750 mg PO TID	5	4	(80.0)	1	(20.0)	0	(0.0)
Metronidazole	750 mg IV TID	1	0	(0.0)	1	(100.0)	0	(0.0)
Pyrimethamine/ sulfa	25 mg PO per day of pyrimethamine	4	4	(100.0)	0	(0.0)	0	(0.0)
Diloxanide furoate	500 mg PO TID	3	2	(66.7)	0	(0.0)	1**	(33.3)
Quinacrine	100 mg PO TID	3	3	(100.0)	0	(0.0)	0	(0.0)
Diiodohydroxyquin	650 mg PO TID	2	2	(100.0)	0	(0.0)	0	(0.0)
Tetracycline	500 mg PO QID	3	1	(33.3)	2	(66.6)	0	(0.0)
Doxycycline	100 mg PO per day	2	2	(100.0)	0	(0.0)	0	(0.0)
Pentamidine	4 mg/kg IM per day	2	2	(100.0)	0	(0.0)	0	(0.0)
Chloroquine/ `primaquine	500 mg PO per day of chloroquine	1	1	(100.0)	0	(0.0)	0	(0.0)

*Some patients received more than one drug.

[†]BID = twice daily; TID = three times daily; QID = four times daily; PO = orally; IV = intravenously

[§]Decrease in number of stools by at least 50%.

[¶]Absence of diarrhea for more than 2 weeks and stool examination negative for *Cryptosporidium*.

**Improvement temporally related to stopping prednisone.

The second patient, who also had a clinical and parasitologic response, subsequently died of PCP. In early February 1982, 6 months before his death, he had onset of watery diarrhea, and a small bowel biopsy showed Cryptosporidium. Treatment with furazolidone (100 mg four times a day) was initiated on May 5, and within 6 days, the patient had gained 1.1 kilograms (3.4 pounds); parenteral nutrition was discontinued, although he continued to produce a liter of watery stool each day. Ten days after treatment was started, his stools became formed for the first time in 4 months, but Cryptosporidium oocysts were still present. Furazolidone was increased to 150 mg four times daily. Twenty days after therapy was starty (10 days after the higher dose of furazolidone was begun), the patient had one bowel movement a day, but his stool was still positive for Cryptosporidium and remained positive despite continued use of furazolidone at 150 mg four times daily for a total of 2 months. At that time, two stool examinations failed to detect oocysts, and the furazolidone was stopped. One week later, the patient developed PCP; despite treatment with trimethoprim-sulfamethoxazole, he died 2 weeks later on July 22. An autopsy was not permitted.

After various treatment regimens, seven patients have had partial or transitory decreases in their diarrhea. Two received no anti-parasitic drugs. A third patient temporarily improved after treatment with furazolidone (100 mg orally four times a day for 7 days), although 2

77

weeks elapsed between the end of treatment with furazolidone and the onset of clinical improvement. The patient's diarrhea abated, but follow-up stool examinations remained positive for Cryptosporidium. Three months after furazolidone therapy, he again developed diarrhea, and his stools were positive for Cryptosporidium. Two patients had less diarrhea when given tetracycline. The first received tetracycline 500 mg orally four times a day for 4 months. His diarrhea decreased from 12 watery stools to three loose stools per day, but stool examination after 4 months of therapy still showed Cryptosporidium. The second patient, given the same treatment, also had a reduction in the number of stools. When the drug was discontinued, his diarrhea again increased.

Two patients' diarrhea stopped following treatment with opiates and metronidazole, given orally in one case and intravenously in the other. Neither patient had diarrhea after a few days of treatment, but both died within 1 week, and autopsies were not allowed. The first patient died from suspected peritonitis; the second died with disseminated Kaposi's sarcoma and pneumonia.

The remaining 12 patients have had continuous, severe diarrhea. In addition to the drugs listed in Table 1, bovine-transfer factor has been given to one patient and intravenous gamma globulin to two patients; neither was effective. At present, 14 (66.7%) of the 21 individuals have died, and six are alive with persistent diarrhea. In no instance was cryptosporidiosis thought to be the direct cause of death, but the associated severe malnutrition was often considered a contributing factor.

Shortly before cryptosporidiosis was recognized in AIDS patients, investigators at the U. S. Department of Agriculture National Animal Disease Center (NADC) began testing drugs for efficacy against Cryptosporidium in animals; results of these initial studies were published in February, 1982(2). More recently, five additional drugs have been evaluated at the NADC. Calves or pigs up to 14 days old without infection were given the drugs orally twice daily. One day after the drugs were started, each animal received a single oral inoculation of Cryptosporidium. The following drugs (with dozes in mg/kg/day) were tested: amprolium (10.7), difluoromethylomithine (1250) plus bleomysin (6 IM), diloxanide furoate (125.0), dimetridazole (19.0), ipronidazole (23.8), lasalocid (0.7), metronidazole (23.8), monensin (4.8), oxytetracycline (50.0), pentamidine (10.0), quinacrine (11.9), salinomycin (6.0), sulfaquinoxaline (200.0), sulfadimidine (119.0), and trimethoprim (4.8) plus sulfadiazine (23.8). Although small numbers of animals were tested in each treatment group, no drugs prevented fecal shedding of oocysts or reduced the number of Cryptosporidium seen on intestinal biopsies.

Reported by J Goldfarb, MD, H Tanowitz, MD, Albert Einstein College of Medicine, Bronx, R Grossman, MD, Medical Arts Center Hospital, C Bonanno, MD, D Kaufman, MD, P Ma, PhD, St Vincent's Medical Center, R Soave, MD, New York Hospital-Cornell Medical Center, D Armstrong, MD, J Gold, MD, Memorial Sloan-Kettering Cancer Center, S Dikman, MD, M Finkel, MD, H Sacks, MD, Mt Sinai Medical Center, R Press, MD, New York University Medical Center, D William, MD, St. Luke's-Roosevelt Hospital, S Friedman, MD, New York City Dept of Health, R Rothenberg, MD, State Epidemiologist, New York State Dept of Health; S Brown, MD, United Hospitals, Newark, WE Parkin, DVM, State Epidemiologist, New Jersey State Dept of Health; EJ Bergquist, MD, Thomas Jefferson University Hospital, Philadelphia, CW Hays, MD, State Epidemiologist, Pennsylvania State Dept of Health; P Forgacs, MD, Lahey Clinic Medical Center, Burlington, L Weinstein, MD, Brigham and Women's Hospital, Boston, NJ Fiumars, MD, State Epidemiologist, Massachusetts State Dept of Public Health; D Busch, MD, San Francisco, M Derezin, MD, M Gottlieb, MD, J Matthew, MD, W Weinstein, MD, UCLA Center for Health Sciences, J Chin, MD, State Epidemiologist, California Dept of Health Svcs; H Moon, PhD, National Animal Disease Center, Ames, Iowa; AIDS Activity, Div of Parasitic Diseases, Center for Infectious Diseases, CDC.

Editorial Note: Cryptosporidium is a protozoan parasite; it is a well recognized cause of diarrhea in animals, especially calves, but has only rarely been associated with diarrhea in humans(3). Individuals with normal immune function who have developed cryptosporidiosis have self-limited diarrhea lasting 1-2 weeks, but immunosuppressed individuals have developed chronic diarrhea. An effective drug to treat cryptosporidiosis has not been identified, and the above reports are equally discouraging. Of seven patients who are still living, only one has no diarrhea at present. His recovery coincided with treatment with diloxanide furoate and discontinuation of prednisone. It seems unlikely that diloxanide furoate was responsible for his recovery, since three other patients who received the drug did not respond, and the drug was ineffective in experimentally infected pigs given nearly six times the recommended human dose. It is similarly difficult to be certain that improvement reported in other patients was due to the drugs they received because only a few patients receiving a drug responded, responses were brief, and the same or similar drugs were ineffective in preventing infection in experimental animals. The difficulty in interpreting isolated responses is underscored by the two patients who improved before any specific therapy began.

Since none of the drugs reported above appears clearly efficacious, additional tests of other anti-parasitic drugs in animals are needed. Until an effective drug for cryptosporidiosis is identified or the underlying immune deficiency in patients with AIDS becomes correctable, management of diarrhea due to cryptosporidiosis will continue to focus on supportive care.

References

1. Anderson BC. Patterns of shedding of cryptosporidial oocysts in Idaho calves. J Am Vet Med Assoc 1981;178:982-4.
2. Moon HW, Woode GN, Ahrens FA. Attempted chemoprophylaxis of cryptosporidiosis in calves. Vet Rec 1982;110:181.
3. CDC. Human cryptosporidiosis — Alabama. MMWR 1982; 31:252-4.

December 10, 1982

Update on Acquired Immune Deficiency Syndrome (AIDS) among Patients with Hemophilia A

In July 1982, three heterosexual hemophilia A patients, who had developed Pneumocystis carinii pneumonia and other opportunistic infections, were reported(1). Each had in vitro evidence of lymphopenia and two patients who were specifically tested had evidence of T-lymphocyte abnormalities. All three have since died. In the intervening 4 months, four additional heterosexual hemophilia A patients have developed one or more opportunistic infections accompanied by in vitro evidence of cellular immune deficiency; these four AIDS cases and one highly suspect case are presented below. Data from inquiries about the patients' sexual activities, drug usage, travel, and residence provide no suggestion that disease could have been acquired through contact with each other, with homosexuals, with illicit drug abusers, or with Haitian immigrants — groups at increased risk for AIDS compared with the general U.S. population. All these patients have received Factor VIII concentrates, and all but one have also received other blood components.

Case 1: A 55-year-old severe hemophiliac from Alabama developed anorexia and progressive weight loss beginning in September 1981. He had developed adult-onset diabetes mellitus in 1973, which had required insulin therapy since 1978. He had had acute hepatitis (type unknown) in 1975. In March 1982, he was hospitalized for herpes zoster and a 17-kg weight loss. Hepatosplenomegaly was noted. The absolute lymphocyte count was 450/mm^3. Liver enzymes were elevated; antibodies to hepatitis B core and surface antigens were present. A liver biopsy showed changes consistent with persistent hepatitis. Evaluation for an occult malignancy was negative. The zoster resolved following 5 days of adenosine arabinoside therapy.

In early June, he was readmitted with fever and respiratory symptoms. Chest x-ray showed bibasilar infiltrates. No causative organism was identified, but clinical improvement occurred coincident with administration of broad spectrum antibiotics. Laboratory studies as an outpatient documented transient thrombocytopenia (63,000/mm^3) and persistent inversion of his T-helper/T-suppressor ratio (T_H/T_S=0.2). He was readmitted for the third time in early September with fever, chills and nonproductive cough. His cumulative weight loss was now 47 kg. Chest x-ray demonstrated bilateral pneumonia, and open lung biopsy showed infection with P. carinii. He responded to sulfamethoxazole/trimethoprim (SMZ/TMP). His T-cell defects persist.

Case 2: A 10-year-old severe hemophiliac from Pennsylvania had been treated with Factor VIII concentrate on a home care program. He had never required blood transfusion. He had been remarkably healthy until September 1982 when he experienced intermitten episodes of fever and vomiting. Approximately 2 weeks later, he also developed persistent anorexia, fatigue, sore throat, and nonproductive cough. On October 20, he was admitted to a hospital with a temperature of 38.4C (101.2F) and a respiratory rate of 60/min. Physical examination revealed cervical adenopathy but no splenomegaly. The absolute number of circulating lymphocytes was low (580/mm^3) and the T-helper/T-suppressor ratio was markedly reduced (T_H/T_S=0.1). His platelet count was 171,000/mm^3. Serum levels of IgG, IgA, and IgM were markedly elevated. Chest x-rays showed bilateral pneumonia and an open lung biopsy revealed massive infiltration with P. carinii and Cryptococcus neoformans. Intravenous SMZ/TMP and amphotericin B have led to marked clinical improvement, but the T-cell abnormalities persist.

Case 3: A 49-year-old patient from Ohio with mild hemophilia had been treated relatively infrequently with Factor VIII concentrate. During the summer of 1982, he noted dysphagia and a weight loss of approximately 7 kg. In October, he was treated for cellulitis of the right hand. Two weeks later, he was observed by a close relative to be dyspneic. He was admitted in November with progressive dyspnea and diaphoresis. Chest x-rays suggested diffuse pneumonitis. His WBC count was 11,000/mm^3 with 9% lymphocytes (absolute lymphocyte number 990/mm^3). The T_H/T_S ratio was 0.25. Open lung biopsy revealed P. carinii. The patient was treated with SMZ/TMP for 6 days with no improvement, and pentamidine isethionate was added. Virus cultures of sputum and chest tube drainage revealed herpes simplex virus. He died on November 22.

Case 4: A 52-year-old severe hemophiliac from Missouri was admitted to a hospital in April 1982 with fever, lymphadenopathy, and abdominal pain. Persistently low numbers of circulating lymphocytes were noted (480/mm^3). Granulomata were seen on histopathologic examination of a bone marrow aspirate. Cultures were positive for Histoplasma capsulatum. The patient improved after therapy with amphotericin B. During the following summer and early fall, he developed fever, increased weight loss, and difficulty thinking. On readmission in early November, he had esophageal candidiasis. Laboratory tests showed profound leukopenia and lymphopenia. A brain scan showed a left frontal mass, which was found to be an organizing hematoma at the time of craniotomy. A chest x-ray showed "fluffy" pulmonary infiltrates. Therapy with SMZ/TMP was begun. Exploratory laparotomy revealed no malignancy. A spenectomy was performed. Biopsies of liver, spleen, and lymph node tissues were negative for H capsulatum granulomata. The lymphoid tissue including the spleen showed an absence of lymphocytes. His total WBC declined to 400/mm^3 and the T_H/T_S cell ratio was 0.1. He died shortly thereafter.

Suspect Case: Described below is an additional highly suspect case that does not meet the strict criteria defining AIDS. A 7-year-old severe hemophilia from Los Angeles had mild mediastinal adenopathy on chest x-ray in September 1981. In March 1982, he developed a spontaneous subdural hematoma requiring surgical evacuation. In July, he developed parotitis. In August, he developed pharyngitis and an associated anterior and posterior cervical adenopathy, which has not resolved. In late September, he developed herpes zoster over the right thigh and buttock, and oral candidiasis. Chest x-rays revealed an increase of the mediastinal adenopathy and the appearance of new perihilar infiltrates. In late October, enlargement of the cervical nodes led to a lymph node biopsy. Architectural features of the node were grossly altered, with depletion of lymphocytes. Heterophile tests were negative. IgG, IgA, and IgM levels were all elevated. He has a marked reduction in T-helper cells and a T_H/T_S ratio equal to 0.4. Recent progressive adenoid enlargement has caused significant upper airway obstruction and resultant sleep apnea.

Reported by M-C Poon, MD, A Landay, PhD, University of Alabama Medical Center, J Alexander, MD, Jefferson County Health Dept, W Birch, MD, State Epidemiologist, Alabama Dept of Health; ME Eyster, MD, H Al-Mondhiry, MD, JO Ballard, MD, Hershey Medical Center, E Witte, VMD, Div of Epidemiology, C Hayes, MD, State Epidemiologist, Pennsylvania State Dept of Health; LO Pass, MD, JP Myers, MD, J Politis, MD, R Goldberg MD, M Bhatti, MD, M Arnold, MD, J York MD, Youngstown Hospital Association, T Halpin, MD, State Epidemiologist, Ohio Dept of Health; L Herwaldt, MD, Washington University Medical Center, A Spivack, MD, Jewish Hospital, St. Louis, HD Donnell MD, State Epidemiologist, Missouri Dept of Health; D Powers, MD, Los Angeles County-University of Southern California Medical Center,

SL Fannin, MD, Los Angeles County Dept of Health Svcs. J Chin, MD, State Epidemiologist, California State Dept of Health; AIDS Activity, Div of Host Factors, Div of Viral Diseases, Center for Infectious Diseases, Field Svcs Div, Epidemiology Program Office, CDC.

Editorial Note: These additional cases of AIDS among hemophilia A patients share several features with the three previously reported cases. All but one are severe hemophiliacs, requiring large amounts of Factor VIII concentrate. None had experienced prior opportunistic infections. All have been profoundly lymphopenix (less than 1000 lymphocytes/mm^3) and have had irreversible deficiencies in T-lymphocytes. Clinical improvement of opportunistic infections with medical therapy has been short lived. Two of the five have died.

In most instances, these patients have been the first AIDS cases in their cities, states, or regions. They have had no known common medications, occupations, habits, types of pets, or any uniform antecedent history of personal or family illnesses with immunological relevance.

Although complete information is not available on brands and lot numbers for the Factor VIII concentrate used by these additional five patients during the past few years, efforts to collect and compare these data with information obtained from the earlier three cases are underway. No common lot numbers has been found among the lots of Factor VIII given to the five patients from whom such information is currently available.

These additional cases provide important perspectives on AIDS in U. S. hemophiliacs. Two of the patients described here are 10 years of age or less, and children with hemophilia must now be considered at risk for the disease. In addition, the number of cases continues to increase, and the illness may pose a significant risk for patients with hemophilia.

The National Hemophilia Foundation and CDC are now conducting a national survey of hemophilia treatment centers to estimate the prevalence of AIDS-associated diseases during the past 5 years and to provide active surveillance of AIDS among patients with hemophilia.

Physicians are encouraged to continue to report AIDS-suspect diseases among hemophilia patients to the CDC through local and state health departments.

Reference

1.   CDC. Pneumocystis carinii pneumonia among persons with hemophilia A. MMWR 1982;31:365-7.

Possible Transfusion-Associated Acquired Immune Deficiency Syndrome (AIDS)
— California

CDC has received a report of a 20-month old infant from the San Francisco area who developed unexplained cellular immunodeficiency and opportunistic infection. This occurred after multiple transfusions, including a transfusion of platelets derived from the blood of a male subsequently found to have the acquired immune deficiency syndrome (AIDS).

The infant, a white male, was delivered by caesarian section on March 3, 1981. The estimated duration of pregnancy was 33 weeks; and the infant weighed 2850 g. The mother was known to have developed Rh sensitization during her first pregnancy, and amniocentesis done during this, her second, pregnancy showed the fetus had erythroblastosis fetalis. The infant had asphyxia at birth and required endotracheal intubation. Because of hyperbilirubinemia, six double-volume exchange transfusions were given over a 4-day period. During the 1-month hospitalization following birth, the infant received blood products, including whole blood, packed red blood cells, and platelets from 19 donors. All blood products were irradiated.

After discharge in April 1981, the infant appeared well, although hepatosplenomegaly was noted at age 4 months. At 7 months, he was hospitalized for treatment of severe otitis media. Oral candidiasis developed following antibiotic therapy and persisted. At 9 months of age, he developed anorexia, vomiting, and then jaundice. Transaminase levels were elevated, and serologic tests for hepatitis A and B viruses and cytomegalovirus were negative; non-A non-B hepatitis was diagnosed.

At 14 months of age, the infant developed neutropenia and an autoimmune hemolytic anemia and thrombocytopenia. Immunologic studies showed elevated serum concentrations of IgG, IgA, and IgM, decreased numbers of T-lymphocytes, and impaired T-cell function in vitro. Following these studies, he was begun on systemic corticosteroid therapy for his hematologic disease. Three months later, a bone marrow sample, taken before steroid therapy began, was positive for Mycobacterium avium-intracellulare. Cultures of urine and gastric aspirate, taken while the infant received steroids, also grew M. avium-intracellulare. The infant is now receiving chemotherapy for his mycobacterial infection. He continues to have thrombocytopenia.

The parents and brother of the infant are in good health. The parents are heterosexual non-Haitians and do not have a history of intravenous drug abuse. The infant had no known personal contact with an AIDS patient.

Investigation of the blood products received by the infant during his first month of life has revealed that one of the 19 donors was subsequently reported to have AIDS. The donor, a 48-year-old white male resident of San Francisco, was apparently in good health when he donated blood on March 10, 1981. Platelets derived from this blood were given to the infant on March 11. Eight months later, the donor complained of fatigue and decreased appetite. On examination, he had right axillary lymphadenopathy, and cotton-wool spots were seen in the retina of the left eye. During the next month, December 1981, he developed fever and severe tachypnea and was hospitalized with biopsy-proven Pneumocystis carinii pneumonia.

Although he improved on antimicrobial therapy and was discharged after a 1-month hospitalization, immunologic studies done in March 1982 showed severe cellular immune dysfunction typical of AIDS. In April 1982, he developed fever and oral candidiasis, and began to lose weight. A second hospitalization, beginning in June 1982, was complicated by Salmonella sepsis, perianal herpes simplex virus infection, encephalitis of unknown etiology, and disseminated cytomegalovirus infection. He died in August 1982.

Reported by A Ammann, MD, M Cowan, MD, D Wara, MD, Dept of Pediatrics, University of California at San Francisco, H Goldman, MD, H Perkins, MD, Irwin Memorial Blood Bank, R Lanzerotti, MD, J Gullett, MD, A Duff, MD, St. Francis Memorial Hospital, S Dritz, MD, City/County Health Dept, San Francisco, J Chin, MD, State Epidemiologist, California State Dept of Health Svcs; Field Svcs Div, Epidemiology Program Office, AIDS Activity, Div of Host Factors, Center for Infectious Diseases, CDC.

Editorial Note: The etiology of AIDS remains unknown, but its reported occurrence among homosexual men, intravenous drug abusers, and persons with hemophilia A(1) suggests it may be caused by an infectious agent transmitted sexually or through exposure to blood or blood products. If the infant's illness described in this report is AIDS, it occurrence following receipt of blood products from a known AIDS case adds support to the infectious-agent hypothesis.

Several features of the infant's illness resemble those seen among adults with AIDS. Hypergammaglobulinemia with T-cell depletion and dysfunction are not typical of any of the well-characterized congenital immunodeficiency syndromes(2), but are similar to abnormalities described in AIDS(3). Disseminated M. avium-intracellulare infection, seen in this infant, is a reported manifestation of AIDS(4). Autoimmune thrombocytopenia, also seen in this infant, has been described among several homosexual men with immune dysfunction typical of AIDS(5). Nonetheless, since there is no definitive laboratory test for AIDS, any interpretation of this infant's illness must be made with caution.

If the platelet transfusion contained an etiologic agent for AIDS, one must assume that the agent can be present in the blood of a donor before onset of symptomatic illness and the incubation period for such illness can be relatively long. This model for AIDS transmission is consistent with findings described in an investigation of a cluster of sexually related AIDS cases among homosexual men in southern California(6).

Of the 788 definite AIDS cases among adults reported thus far to CDC, 42 (5.3%) belong to no known risk group (i.e., they are not known to be homosexually active men, intravenous drug abusers, Haitians, or hemophiliacs). Two cases received blood products within 2 years of the onset of their illnesses and are currently under investigation.

This report and continuing reports of AIDS among persons with hemophilia A(7) raise serious questions about the possible transmission of AIDS through blood and blood products. The Assistant Secretary for Health is convening an advisory committee to address these questions.

References

1. CDC. Update on acquired immune deficiency syndrome (AIDS) — United States. MMWR 1982;31:507-8,513-4.
2. Stiehm ER, Fulginiti VA, eds. Immunologic disorders in infants and children. 2nd edition. Philadelphia: WB Saunders Company, 1980.
3. Gottlieb MS, Schroff R, Schanker HM, et al. Pneumocystis carinii pneumonia and mucosal candidiasis in previously healthy homosexual men: evidence of a new acquired cellular immunodeficiency. N Engl J Med 1981;305:1425-31.
4. Greene JB, Sidhu GS, Lewin S, et al. Mycobacterium avium-intracellulare: a cause of disseminated life-threatening infection in homosexuals and drug abusers. Ann Intern Med 1982;97:539-46.
5. Morris L. Distenfeld A, Amorosi E, Karpatkin S. Autoimmune thrombocytopenic purpura in homosexual men. Ann Intern Med 1982; 96(Part 1):714-7.
6. CDC. A cluster of Kaposi's sarcoma and Pneumocystis carinii pneumonia among homosexual male residents of Los Angeles and Orange Counties, California. MMWR 1982;31:305-7.
7. CDC. Update on acquired immune deficiency syndrome (AIDS) among patients with hemophilia A. MMWR 1982;31:644-6, 652.

December 17, 1982

Unexplained Immunodeficiency and Opportunistic Infections in Infants — New York, New Jersey, California

CDC has received reports of four infants (under 2 years of age) with unexplained cellular immunodeficiency and opportunistic infections.

Case 1: The infant, a black/hispanic male weighing 5 lb 14 oz, was born in December 1980 following a 36-38-week pregnancy. Pregnancy has been complicated by bleeding in the fourth month and by preeclampsia in the ninth month. The infant was well until 3 months of age, when oral candidiasis was noted. At 4 months, hepatosplenomegaly was observed, and at 7 months, he had staphylococcal impetigo. Growth, which had been slow, stopped at 9 months. Head circumference, which had been below the third percentile, also stopped increasing. At 9 months, serum levels of IgG and IgA were normal; IgM was high-normal. T-cell studies were normal, except for impaired in-vitro responses to Candida antigen and alloantigen.

At 17 months of age, the infant had progressive pulmonary infiltrates, as well as continuing oral condidiasis, and was hospitalized. Mycobacterium avium-intracellulare was cultured from sputum and bone marrow samples. A CAT scan of the head revealed bilateral calcification of the basal ganglia and subcortical regions of the frontal lobes. Repeat immunologic studies done at age 20 months showed lymphopenia, decreased numbers of T-lymphocytes, and severely impaired T-cell function in vitro; immunoglobulin determinations are pending. The infant remains alive and is receiving therapy for his mycobacterial infection.

The infant's mother, a 29-year-old resident of New York City, gave a history of intravenous drug abuse. Although she was in apparently good health at the time of the infant's birth, she developed fever, dyspnea, and oral candidiasis in October 1981. One month later, she was hospitalized and died of biopsy-proven Pneumocystis carinii pneumonia (PCP). She had been lymphopenic during the hospitalization; further immunologic studies were not done. At autopsy, no underlying cause for immune deficiency was found.

Case 2: The infant, a Haitian male weighing 6 lb 11 oz, was born in January 1981 following full-term pregnancy. The immediate postpartum period was complicated by respiratory distress. Diarrhea developed at 2 weeks of age and persisted. His physical development was retarded. At 5 months, he was hospitalized because of fever and diarrhea. On examination, he had hepatosplenomegaly, lymphadenopathy, and otitis media. While on antibiotics, he developed pulmonary infiltrates. An open lung biopsy revealed Pneumocystis carinii, Cryptococcus neoformans, and cytomegalovirus. Serum IgG, IgA, and IgM concentrations were elevated. The percentage of T-lymphocytes was decreased, but T-cell response to mitogens was normal. The infant died of respiratory insufficiency at 7½ months of age. At autopsy, the thymus, spleen, and lymph nodes showed lymphocyte depletion. His parents were residents of Brooklyn, New York; their health status is unknown.

Case 3: The infant, a Haitian male weighing 8 lb, was born in November 1982 following a normal, full-term pregnancy. He was apparently healthy until 5 months of age, when he was hospitalized with fever and respiratory distress. On examination, he had hepatosplenomegaly. A chest x-ray showed bilateral pulmonary infiltrates. Despite antibiotic therapy, the infant's condition deteriorated, and an open lung biopsy revealed PCP. Immunologic studies showed elevated serum concentrations of IgG, IgA and IgM, decreased percentage of T-lymphocytes, and impaired T-cell function in vitro. The infant died in May 1982. At autopsy, no cardiovascular anomalies were seen; the thymust was hypoplastic, but all lobes were present. His parents were residents of Newark, New Jersey; their health status is unknown.

Case 4: The infant, a white female weighing 5 lb, was born in April 1982 following a normal 35-week pregnancy. She was well until 2 months of age, when oral and vaginal Candida infections were noted. She responded to antifungal therapy, but at 5 months, candidiasis recurred, and she had hepatosplenomegaly. Immunologic evaluation showed that serum IgG, IgA, and IgM levels, normal at 2 months, were now elevated. The percentage of T-lymphocytes was decreased, and lymphocyte response to alloantigen was impaired. At 6 months of age, the infant was hospitalized because of fever and cough. Open lung biopsy revealed PCP. Despite appropriate antibiotic therapy, she died in November 1982.

The infant's mother, a 29-year-old resident of San Francisco, is a prostitute and intravenous drug abuser with a history of oral candidiasis and mild lymphopenia. She has had two other female children by different fathers. These half-sisters also have unexplained cellular immunodeficiency; one died of PCP. The children had not lived together.

None of the four infants described in the case reports was known to have received blood or blood products before onset of illness.

Other cases with opportunistic infections: Six additional young children with opportunistic infections (five with PCP, one with M. avium-intracellulare) and unusual cellular immunodeficiencies are under investigation. Three are male. All six children have died. One was a half-sister of the infant in Case 4.

Other cases without opportunistic infections: Physicians from New York City, New Jersey, and California have reported another 12 young children with immunodeficiencies similar to those seen in cases 1-4 but without life-threatening opportunistic infections. One is the other half-sister of the infant in Case 4. All the children are living; their ages range from 1 to 4 years. Eight are male, Clinical features seen in these 12 infants include: failure to thrive (83%), oral candidiasis (50%), hepatosplenomegaly (92%), generalized lymphadenopathy (92%), and chronic pneumonitis without a demonstrable infection (83%). Of the nine mothers for whom information is available, seven are reported to be intravenous drug abusers. None is Haitian.

Reported by R O'Reilly, MD, D Kirkpatrick, MD, Memorial Sloan-Kettering Cancer Center, C Butkus Small, MD, R Klein, MD, H Keltz, MD, G Friedland, MD, Montefiore Hospital and Medical Center, K Bromberg, MD, S Fikrig, MD, H Mendez, MD, State University of New York, Downstate Medical Center, A Rubinstein, MD, Albert Einstein College of Medicine, M Hollander, MD, Misericordia Hospital Medical Center, F Siegal, MD, Mt Sinai School of Medicine, J Greenspan, MD, NOrthshore University Hospital, M Lange, MD, St Lukes-Roosevelt Hospital Center, S Friedman, MD, New York City Dept of Health, R Rothenberg, MD, State Epidemiologist, New York State Dept of Health; J Oleske, MD, C Thomas MD, R Guerrero, MD, B Mojica, MD, W Parkin, DVM, State Epidemiologist, New Jersey State Dept of Health; M Cowan, MD, A Ammann, MD, D Wara, MD, University of California at San Francisco, S Dritz, MD, City/County Health Dept, San Francisco, J Chin, MD, State Epidemiologist, California State Dept of Health Svcs; Field Svcs Div, Epidemiology Program Office, AIDS Activity, Div of Host Factors, Center for Infectious Diseases, CDC.

Editorial Note: The nature of the immune dysfunction described in the four case reports is unclear. The infants lacked the congenital anomalies associated with Di George's syndrome. The immunologic features of high-normal or elevated immunoglobulin levels and T-lymphocyte depletion are not typical of any of the well-defined congenital immunodeficiency syndromes. They have, however, been described in a few children with variants of Nezelof's syndrome, a rare, poorly characterized illness of unknown etiology[1,2]. The occurrence of immune deficiency in the infant in case 4 and in her half-sisters raises the possibility of an inherited disorder. However, inheritance would have to have occurred in a dominant manner, an inheritance pattern not previously described for immunodeficiency resembling that seen in these half-sisters.

It is possible that these infants had the acquired immune deficiency syndrome (AIDS). Although the mother of the infant in case 1 was not studied immunologically, her death from PCP was probably secondary to AIDS. The mothers of the other three infants were Haitian or intravenous drug abusers, groups at increased risk for AIDS[3]. The immunologic features described in the case reports resemble those seen both in adults with AIDS[4] and in a child reported to have developed immunodeficiency following receipt of blood products from a patient with AIDS[5]. Case 2 had essentially normal T-cell responses to mitogens in vitro. This finding is atypical for AIDS, but it has been seen in a few adult AIDS cases[6].

82

Although the etiology of AIDS remains unknown, a series of epidemiologic observations suggests it is caused by an infectious agent (3,5,7-9). If the infants described in the four case reports had AIDS, exposure to the putative "AIDS agent" must have occurred very early. Cases 2-4 were less than 6 months old when they had serious opportunistic infections. Case 1 has oral candidiasis beginning at 3 months of age, although M. avium-intracellulare infection was not documented until 17 months. Transmission of an "AIDS agent" from mother to child, either in utero or shortly after birth, could account for the early onset of immunodeficiency in these infants.

The relationship between the illnesses seen in the reported cases with severe opportunistic infection and the 12 infants without such infections is unclear at present. The immune dysfunction seen in the children and the sociodemographic profiles of the mothers appear similar in both groups. Prospective study of the 12 children is necessary to define the natural history of their illnesses and the possible relationship of their illnesses to AIDS.

References

1. Lawlor GJ, Jr. Ammann AJ, Wright WC, Jr, La Franchi SH, Bilstrom D, Stiehm ER. The syndrome of cellular immunodeficiency with immunoglobulins. J Pediatr 1974;84:183-92.
2. Ammann AJ, Hong R. Disorders of the T-cell system. In: Stiehm ER, Fulginiti VA, eds. Immunologic disorders in infants and children. 2nd ed. Philadelphia: Saunders 1980:286-348.
3. CDC. Update on acquired immune deficiency syndrome (AIDS) — United States. MMWR 1982;31:507-8, 513-4.
4. Gottlieb MS, Schroff R, Schanker HM, et al. Pneumocystis carinii pneumonia and mucosal candidiasis in previously healthy homosexual men: evidence of a new acquired cellular immunodeficiency. N Engl J Med 1981;305:1425-31.
5. CDC. Possible transfusion-associated acquired immune deficiency syndrome (AIDS) — California. MMWR 1982;31:652-4.
6. CDC. Unpublished data.
7. CDC. A cluster of Kaposi's sarcoma and Pneumocystis carinii pneumonia among homosexual male residents of Los Angeles and Orange Counties, California. MMWR 1982;31:305-7.
8. CDC. Pneumocystis carinii pneumonia among persons with hemophilia A. MMWR 1982;31:365-7.
9. CDC. Update on acquired immune deficiency syndrome (AIDS) among patients with hemophilia A. MMWR 1982;31:644-6, 652.

January 7, 1983

Immunodeficiency among Female Sexual Partners of Males with Acquired Immune Deficiency Syndrome (AIDS) — New York

CDC has received reports of two females with cellular immunodeficiency who have been steady sexual partners of males with the acquired immune deficiency syndrome (AIDS).

Case 1: A 37-year-old black female began losing weight and developed malaise in June 1982. In July, she had oral candidiasis and generalized lymphadenopathy and then developed fever, non-productive cough, and diffuse intestinal pulmonary infiltrates. A transbronchial biopsy revealed Pneumocystis carinii pneumonia (PCP). Immunologic studies showed elevated immunoglobulin levels, lymphopenia, and an undetectable number of T-helper cells. She responded to antimicrobial therapy, but 3 months after hospital discharge had lymphadenopathy, oral candidiasis, and persistent depletion of T-helper cells.

The patient had no previous illnesses or therapy associated with immunosuppression. She admitted to moderate alcohol consumption, but denied intravenous (IV) drug abuse. Since 1976, she had lived with and had been the steady sexual partner of a male with a history of IV drug abuse. He developed oral candidiasis in March 1982 and in June had PCP. He had laboratory evidence of immune dysfunction typical of AIDS and died in November 1982.

Case 2: A 23-year-old Hispanic female was well until February 1982 when she developed generalized lymphadenopathy. Immunologic studies showed elevated immunoglobulin levels, lymphopenia, decreased T-helper cell numbers, and a depressed T-helper/T-suppressor cell ratio (0.82). Common infectious causes of lymphadenopathy were excluded by serologic testing. A lymph node biopsy showed lymphoid hyperplasia. The lymphadenopathy has persisted for almost a year; no etiology for it has been found.

The patient had no previous illnesses or therapy associated with immunosuppression and denied IV drug abuse. Since the summer of 1981, her only sexual partner has been a bisexual male who denied IV drug abuse. He developed malaise, weight loss and lymphadenopathy in June 1981 and oral candidiasis and PCP in June 1982. Skin lesions, present for 6 months, were biopsied in June 1982 and diagnosed as Kaposi's sarcoma. He has laboratory evidence of immune dysfunction typical of AIDS and remains alive.

Reported by C Harris, MD, C Butkus Small, MD, G Friedland, MD, R Klein, MD, B Moll, PhD, E Emeson, MD, I Spigland, MD, N Steigbigel, MD, Depts of Medicine and Pathology, Montefiore Medical Center, North Central Bronx Hospital, and Albert Einstein College of Medicine, R Reiss, S Friedman, MD, New York City Dept of Health, R Rothenberg, MD, State Epidemiologist, New York State Dept of Health; AIDS Activity, Center for Infectious Diseases, CDC.

Editorial Note: Each reported female patient developed immunodeficiency during a close relationship, including repeated sexual contact, with a male who had AIDS. Patient 1 fits the CDC case definition of AIDS used for epidemiologic surveillance(1). Patient 2 does not meet this definition, but her persistent, generalized lymphadenopathy and cellular immunodeficiency suggest a syndrome described among homosexual men(2). The epidemiologic and immunologic features of this "lymphadenopathy syndrome" and the progression of some patients with this syndrome to Kaposi's sarcoma and opportunistic infections suggest it is part of the AIDS spectrum(3,4). Other than their relationships with their male sexual partners, neither patient had any apparent risk factor for AIDS. Both females specifically denied IV drug abuse.

Epidemiologic observations increasingly suggest that AIDS is caused by an infectious agent. The description of a cluster of sexually related AIDS patients among homosexual males in southern California suggested that such an agent could be transmitted sexually or through other intimate contact(5). AIDS has also been reported in both members of a male homosexual couple in Denmark(6). The present report supports the infectious-agent hypothesis and the possibility that transmission of the putative "AIDS agent" may occur among both hetero-sexual and male homosexual couples.

Since June 1981, CDC has received reports of 43 previously healthy females who have developed PCP or other opportunistic infections typical of AIDS. Of these 43 patients, 13 were reported as neither Haitians nor IV drug abusers. One of these 13 females is described in case 1; another four, including two wives, are reported to be steady sexual partners of male IV drug abusers. Although none of the four male partners has had an overt illness suggesting AIDS, immunologic studies of blood specimens from one of these males have shown abnormalities of lymphoproliferative response(7). Conceivably, these male drug abusers are carriers of an infectious agent that has not made them ill but caused AIDS in their infected female sexual partners.

References

1. CDC. Update on acquired immune deficiency syndrome (AIDS) — United States. MMWR 1982;31:507-8, 513-4.

2. CDC. Persistent, generalized lymphadenopathy among homosexual males. MMWR 1982;31:249-51.

3. Mathur U, Enlow RW, Spigland I, William DC, Winchester RJ, Mildvan D. Generalized lymphadenopathy: a prodrome of Kaposi's sarcoma in male homosexuals? Abstract. Twenty-second Interscience Conference on Antimicrobial Agents and Chemotherapy. Miami Beach, Florida. October 4-6, 1982.

4. CDC. Unpublished data.

5. CDC. A cluster of Kaposi's sarcoma and Pneumocystis carinii pneumonia among homosexual males residents of Los Angeles and Orange counties, California. MMWR 1982;31:305-7.

6. Gerstoft J. Malchow-Moller A, Bygbjerg I, et al. Severe acquired immunodeficiency in European homosexual men. Br Med J 1982; 285:17-9.

7. Masur H, Michelis MA, Wormser GP, et al. Opportunistic infection in previously healthy women, initial manifestations of a community-acquired cellular immunodeficiency. Ann Intern Med 1982;97:533-9.

January 7, 1983

Acquired Immune Deficiency Syndrome (AIDS) in Prison Inmates
— New York, New Jersey

CDC has received reports from New York and New Jersey of 16 prison inmates with the acquired immune deficiency syndrome (AIDS).

New York: Between November 1981 and October 1982, ten AIDS cases (nine with Penumocystis carinii pneumonia [PCP] and one with Kaposi's sarcoma [KS] were reported among inmates of New York State correctional facilities. The patients had been imprisoned from 3 to 36 months (mean 18.5 months) before developing symptoms of these two diseases.

All ten patients were males ranging in age from 23 to 38 years (mean 29.7 years). Four were black, and of the six who were white, two were Hispanic. Four of the nine patients with PCP died; the patient with KS is alive. All nine patients with PCP also developed oral candidiasis. None of the patients was known to have an underlying illness associated with immunosuppression, and no such illness was found at postmortem examination of the four patients who died. PCP was diagnosed in all nine cases by means of transbronchial or open-lung biopsy, while KS was diagnosed by biopsy of a lesion on the leg.

Evidence of cellular immune dysfunction was present in the nine patients with PCP: eight were lymphopenic, and all nine were anergic to multiple cutaneous recall antigens. An abnormally low ratio of T-helper to T-suppressor cells was present in six of seven patients tested, and in vitro lymphocyte proliferative responses to a variety of mitogens and antigens were significantly depressed or negative in the six patients tested. The one patient with KS had cutaneous anergy and a decreased proportion of T-cells in his peripheral blood. The ratio of T-helper to T-suppressor cells was normal; studies of lymphoproliferative response were not done.

All ten patients reported that they were heterosexual before imprisonment; one is known to have had homosexual contacts since confinement. However, the nine patients with PCP were regular users of intravenous (IV) drugs (principally heroin and cocaine) in New York City before imprisonment. The seven patients who were extensively interviewed denied regular IV drug use since confinement, although two reported occasional use of IV drugs while in prison. The ten patients were housed in seven different prisons when they first developed PCP or KS. Three patients who developed symptoms of PCP within 1 month of each other were confined in the same facility. However, they were housed in separate buildings, and each denied any social interaction (including homosexual contact and drug use) with the other patients.

All inmates of the New York State correctional system receive a medical evaluation when transferred from local or county jails; this usually includes a leukocyte count. Of the nine AIDS patients who initially had leukocyte counts, seven did not then have symptoms of

84

AIDS. Four of these seven asymptomatic males had leukocyte counts below 4000/mm^3. For these four, the time between leukocyte counts and development of clinical PCP symptoms ranged from 4 to 19 months (mean 11.5 months).

New Jersey: Of the 48 AIDS cases reported from New Jersey since June 1981, six have involved inmates of New Jersey correctional facilities. All six had PCP. They were imprisoned from 1 to 36 months (mean 17.5 months) before onset of symptoms.

All six patients were males ranging in age from 26 to 41 years (mean 32 years). Three were black; three, white. Four of the six died within 1-8 months of onset of their illnesses. None of the six was known to have underlying illness associated with immune deficiency. Immunologic studies of the two survivors have shown cutaneous anergy, leukopenia, lymphopenia, and increased circulating immune complexes. T-cell studies were not done.

All six patients have histories of chronic IV drug abuse. Of the five for whom sexual orientation was reported, four were heterosexual, and one was homosexual. The two living patients have denied both IV drug use and homosexual activity since imprisonment. No two of the six patients have been confined in the same facility at the same time.

Reported by: G Wormser, MD, F Duncanson, MD, L Krupp, MD, Dept of Medicine, Westchester County Medical Center, R Tomar, MD, Dept of Pathology, Upstate Medical Center, DM Shah, MD, Horton Memorial Hospital, B Maguire, G Gavis, MD, New York State Dept of Corrections, W Gaunay, J Lawrence, J Wasser, Medical Review Board, New York State Commission of Corrections, D Morse, MD, New York State Bureau of Communicable Disease Control, R Rothenberg, MD, State Epidemiologist, New York State Dept of Health; P Vieux, MD, K Vacarro, RN, St. Francis Hospital, R Reed, MD, A Koenigfest, New Jersey State Dept of Corrections, I Guerrero, MD, W Parkin, DVM, State Epidemiologist, New Jersey State Dept of Health; Field Svcs Div, Epidemiology Program Office, Div of Host Factors and AIDS Activity, Center for Infectious Diseases, CDC.

Editorial Note: Since male homosexuals and IV drug abusers are known to be at increased risk for AIDS[1], the occurrence of AIDS among imprisoned members of these groups might have been anticipated. Increasingly, epidemiologic observations suggest that AIDS is caused by an infectious agent transmitted sexually or through exposure to blood or blood products. Because of the difficulties inherent in interviewing prisoners, data elicited in such interviews must be viewed cautiously. Given this caution, the histories obtained from the inmates indicate that all or most of their drug use, and, by inference, their exposure to a blood-borne agent, occurred before confinement.

The presence of leukopenia in some of the prisoners tested on admission to the prison system may imply that laboratory evidence of immune dysfunction may precede clinical illness by months.

Health care personnel for correctional facilities should be aware of the occurrence of AIDS in prisoners, particularly prisoners with histories of IV drug abuse. AIDS cases identified in prisoners should be reported to local and state correctional and health departments and to CDC.

Reference
1. CDC. Update on acquired immune deficiency syndrome (AIDS) — United States. MMWR 1982;31:507-8, 513-4.

APPENDIX D

A.I.D.S.: A SCIENTIFIC AND CLINICAL BIBLIOGRAPHY

compiled by Richard B. Pearce, Ph.D.
with editorial assistance from Gary Babcock

Reprinted by permission of
Kaposi's Sarcoma Research and Education Foundation
P. O. Box 14227
San Francisco, California 94114
(415) 864-4376
First Edition
March, 1983

A.I.D.S.: A SCIENTIFIC AND CLINICAL BIBLIOGRAPHY

Community Acquired Immunodeficiency State and Diseases in Homosexual Men, Haitians, IV-Drug Users, Prisoners, Hemophiliacs, Infants and Others

Alteras, I., et al., 1981. The high incidence of Tinea pedis and Unguim in patients with Kaposi's Sarcoma. MYCOPATHOLOGIA 74(3):177-179.

Auerbach, D.M., Bennet, J.V., Brachman, P.S. et al., 1982. Epidemiological aspects of the current outbreak of Kaposi's sarcoma and opportunistic infections. NEW ENG. J. MED. 306-248-252.

Babb, R.R., 1979. Sexually transmitted infections in homosexual men. POSTGRADUATE MEDICINE 63(3):215-218.

Bannister, B., 1982. Hepatitis in homosexual men: possibility of urinary transmission. BRITISH MED. J. 285(July 17):223-224.

Bart, R.S., et al., 1982. Tumor conference 41: Spontaneously disappearing Kaposi's sarcoma. JOURNAL OF DERMATOLOGIC SURGERY AND ONCOLOGY 8(4):257-259.

Bolan, R., 1981. Sexually transmitted diseases in homosexuals: focusing the attack. SEXUALLY TRANS-MITTED DISEASES 8(4):293-297.

Borkorvik, S., et al., 1981. Kaposi's Sarcoma presenting in the homosexual man: A new and striking phenomenon. ARIZONA MED. 38(12):902-904.

Brennan, R.O., Durack, D.T., 1981. Gay Compromise Syndrome. LANCET Dec. 12 II(8259):1338-1339.

Brenner, S., Krakowski, A. Schewach-Millet, M. et al. 1982. increased frequency of HLA-Aw19 in Kaposi's sarcoma. TISSUE ANTIGENS 19:392-394.

Beurey, J., Mazet, J., de Ren, G., Vaillant, G., 1976 Association maladie de kaposi — maladie de Hodgkin. ANN DERMATOL. SYPHILO. (PARIS) 103:151-159.

Brunning, R.D., Foley, J.F., Fortuny, I.E., 1963. Hodgkins disease and Kaposi's sarcoma. ARCH. INTER. MED. 112:363-369.

Canadian Medical Association Journal 1982. Acquired immunodeficiency disease syndromes in Canada. CMAJ 127-1161 (Dec. 15).

Centers for Disease Control 1982. Persistent, generalized lymphadenopathy among homosexual males. MMWR 31(19):249-251.

———— 1982. Diffuse, undifferentiated non-Hodgkis lymphoma among homosexual males — United States. MMWR 31(21):277-284.

———— 1982. Update on Kaposi's sarcoma and opportunistic infections in previously healthy persons — United States. MMWR 31(21):294-301.

————— 1982. A cluster of Kaposi's sarcoma and Pneumocystis carinii Pneumonia among homosexual male residents of Los Angeles and Orange Counties, Calif. MMWR 31(23):305-307.

————— 1982. Opportunistic infections and Kaposi's sarcoma among Haitians in the United States MMWR 31(26):353-354.

————— 1982. Pneumocystis carinii pneumonia among persons with hemophilia A. MMWR 31(27): 365-369.

————— 1982. Update on acquired immune deficiency syndrome (A.I.D.S.) United States. MMWR 31(37):507-514.

————— 1982. Acquired Immune Deficiency Syndrome (A.I.D.S.): precautions for clinical and laboratory staffs. MMWR 31(43):577-580.

————— 1982. Cryptosporidiosis: Assessment of Chemotherapy of Males with Acquired Immune Deficiency Syndrome (A.I.D.S.) MMWR 31(44):589-591.

Clemmensen, J. 1982. Kaposi's sarcoma in homosexual men: is it a new disease? (an editorial reply). LANCET II(8288):51-52; July 3.

Comfort, A., 1982. Homosexual practices and immune deficits. LANCET I(8286):1422; June 19.

Conant, M., Volberding, P., Fletcher, V. et al., 1982. Squamous Cell carcinoma in sexual partner of Kaposi's sarcoma patient. LANCET Jan. 30, I(8266):286.

Cooper, H. S., Patchefsky, A.S. et al., 1979. Cloacogenic carcinoma of the anorectum in homosexual men: an observation of four cases. DISEASES OF THE COLON AND RECTUM 22(8):557-558.

Costa, Jose, and Rabson, Alan S., 1983. Generalized Kaposi's sarcoma is not a neoplasm. LANCET I (8314/5):58; Jan1/8.

Coutinho, E.M., 1982. Kaposi's sarcoma and the use of estrogen by male homosexuals. LANCET I:1326 June 12.

Dahling, J.R., Weiss, N.S., et al., 1982. Correlates of homosexual behavior and the incidence of anal cancer. JAMA 247(14):1988-1990.

Darrow, William, Barrett, D., Karla, J. et al., 1981. The gay report on sexually transmitted diseases. AMERICAN J. OF PUBLIC HEALTH 71(9):1004-1011.

Desforges, J.F. 1983. A.I.D.S. and preventive treatment in hemophilia. NEW ENGL. J. MED. 308(2): 94 (Jan. 13).

DeStefano, E. Freidman, R.M., Freidman-Kien, et al., 1982. Acid labile human leukocyte interferon in homosexual men with Kaposi's sarcoma and lymphadenopathy. J. OF INFECTIOUS DISEASES 146(4):451-455.

de Thuin, R., 1982. A.I.D.S. Pilot Study (Mt. Sinai Medical Center, NY) NEW YORK NATIVE 49:11 Oct. 25-Nov. 7.

DeWys, William, Curran, J., Werner, H., et al., 1982. Workshop on Kaposi's sarcoma: meeting report. CANCER TREATMENT REPORTS 66(6):1387-1390.

DiGiovanna, John J., Safai, B. 1981. Kaposi's sarcoma: A retrospective study of 90 cases with particular emphasis on the familial occurrence, ethnic background and prevalence of other diseases. AMERICAN J. MEDICINE 71(5):779-783.

Dobozy, A., Hesz, S. et al., 1973. Immune deficiencies and Kaposi's sarcoma. LANCET II(7829):625 (Sept. 15).

Doherty, J., 1982. PNEUMOCYSTIS CARINII pneumonia in a homosexual male. CANADA DISEASES WEEKLY REPORT 8(13):65-68.

Doll, D.C., List, A.F., 1982. Burkitt's lymphoma in a homosexual. LANCET I (8279):1026-1027 (May 1).

90

Drew, W.L., Miner, R., Ziegler, J., et al., 1982 Cytomegalovirus and Kaposi's sarcoma in young homosexual men. J. INFECT. DISEASE 143:188-192.

Dritz, S. Ainsworth, T.E. et al., 1977. Patterns of sexually transmitted enteric diseases in a city. LANCET II (8027):3-4 (July 2).

Dritz, S. 1980. Medical Aspects of Homosexuality. NEW ENGL. J. MED. 302(8):463-464.

du Bois R.M., Branthwaite, M.A. et al., 1981. Primary PNEUMOCYSTIS CARINII pneumonia and cytomegalovirus infections. LANCET II (8259):1339 (Dec. 12).

Dunk, A., Jenkins, W.J. and S. Sherlock. 1982. Guillaine-Barre syndrome associated with hepatitis A in a male homosexual. BR. J. VENER. DIS. 58:269:270.

Durack, David J. 1981. Opportunistic infections and Kaposi's sarcoma in homosexual men. NEW ENGL. J. MED. 305:1465-1467.

Egbert, P., Pollard, R., et al., 1980. Cytomegalovirus retinitis in immunosuppressed hosts. II. Ocular manifestations. ANNALS OF INTERNAL MED. 93:664.

Epstein, D.M. Gefter, W.B. et al., 1982. Lung disease in homosexual men. RADIOLOGY 143(1):7-10.

Fainstein, V., Bolivar, R., Mavligit, G et al., 1982. Disseminated infection due to MYCOBACTERIUM AVIUM-INTRACELLULARE in a homosexual man with Kaposi's sarcoma. J. OF INFECTIOUS DISEASES 145(4):586.

Fauci, S. 1982. The syndrome of Kaposi's sarcoma and opportunistic infections: an epidemiologically restricted disorder of immunoregulation. ANNALS OF INTERNAL MED. 96(ptl):777-779.

Felman, Y.M. 1980. Homosexual hazards. PRACTIONER 2241349):1151-1156.

Fisher, Y.M., et al., 1980. Kaposi's sarcoma of the base of the tongue. J. OF LARYNGOLOGY AND OTOLOGY 94(6):663-668.

Flegel, K.M., Simard, M., Jessamine, A.G. 1982. Opportunistic infections in a Haitian immigrant — Quebeck. CANADA DISEASES WEEKLY REPORT 8(40):197-199.

Fluker, J.L., 1976. A ten-year study of homosexually transmitted infection. BR. J. VENER. DIS. 52: 155-160.

Fluker, J.L., 1981. Homosexuality and sexually transmitted diseases. BRITISH JOURNAL OF HOSPITAL MEDICINE 26(3):265-266.

Follansbee, S. E., Busch, D., Wofsy, C. B., et al., 1982. An outbreak of Pneumocystis carinii pneumonia in homosexual men. ANNALS OF INTERNAL MED. 96 (ptl):705-713.

Frederick, P., L., Osborn, D., and Cronin, C.M., 1982. Anorectal squamous carcinoma in two homosexual men. LANCET II (8294):391, Aug. 14.

Friedman, A., Freeman, W., Orellana, J., et al., 1982. Cytomegalovirus retinitis and immunodeficiency in homosexual males. LANCET I (8278):958; 1982.

Friedman—Kien, A.E., 1981 Disseminated Kaposi-like sarcoma in young homosexual men. J. AMER. ACAD. DERMATOL. 1981(5):468-470.

Friedman-Kien, Alvin. E., Laubenstein, L.J., Rubenstein, P., et al. 1982. Disseminated Kaposi's sarcoma in Homosexual men. ANNALS OF INTERNAL MEDICINE 96 (6, ptl):693-700.

Frizzera, G. Moran, E.M. et al., 1974. Angio-immunoblastic lymphadenopathy with dysproteinemia. LANCET I (7866):1070-1073.

Gardiner, R., 1982. Acquired Immunodeficiency in homosexual men. RADIOLOGY 143(1):280.

Gardiner, R.B., 1982. Incidence of nodular lymphoid hyperplasia in homosexual men. AMERICAN JOURNAL OF ROENTGENOLOGY 138(3):593.

Geerling, J., 1982. Acquired immunodeficiency and Kaposi's sarcoma in homosexual men. NEDERLANDS TIJDSCHRIFT VOOR GENEESKUNDE 126(14):631-633.

Gerstoft, J. et al., 1982. Severe acquired immunodeficiency in European homosexual men. BRITISH MED. J. 285:17-19.

Gilkey, F. W., 1982. Opportunistic infections and Kaposi's sarcoma in homosexual men. NEW ENGL. J. MED. 306:933; April 15.

Giron, J.A., Martinez, S., and Walzer, P.D., 1982. Should inpatients with Pneumocystis carinii be isolated? LANCET II (8288); July 3.

Goodwin, J.D., et al., 1982. Fatal pneumocystis pneumonia, cryptococosis, and Kaposi's sarcoma in homosexual men. AMERICAN J. OF ROENTGENOLOGY 138(3):580-581.

Gold, K.D., Louys, T., Garrett, T.J. 1982. Aggressive Kaposi's sarcoma in a heterosexual drug addict. NEW ENGL. J. MED. 307(8):498 (Aug. 19).

Goldbaum, J. et al., 1979. Gay bowel Syndrome. MEDICAL J. OF AUSTRALIA 2(13):699 Dec. 29).

Gomez, J., 1981. Homosexuality and sexually transmitted diseases. BRITISH J. OF HOSPITAL MEDICINE 26(6):654 (Dec. 1981).

Goode, E., Troiden, R.R., 1979. Amyl nitrite use in homosexual men. AMERICAN J. OF PSYCHIATRY. 136(8):1067-1069.

Gorin, I. et al., 1982. Kaposi's sarcoma without the U.S. or "popper" connection. LANCET I (8277): 908 (April 17).

Gottlieb, M.S., Ragaz, A., Vogel, J.V., et al., 1981. A preliminary communication on extensively disseminated Kaposi's sarcoma in young homosexual men. AM. J. DERMATOPATH. 3(2)111-114.

Gottlieb, M.S., Schroff, R., Schanker, H.M., et al., 1981. PNEUMOCYSTIS CARINII pneumonia and mucosal candidiasis in previously healthy adult homosexual men. NEW ENGL. J. MED. 305: 1425-1431. (Dec. 10).

Greene, J., Sidhu, G., et al., 1982. MYCOBACTERIUM AVIUMINTRACELLULARE: a cause of disseminated life-threatening infection in homosexuals and drug abusers. ANNALS OF INTER. MED. 97(4):539-546.

Greenberg, Frank, Englow, R., 1982. Screening for risk of Acquired Immune-deficiency syndrome. NEW ENGL. J. MED 307(24):1521.

Groopman, J.E., Gottlieb, M.S., 1982. Kaposi's sarcoma: an oncological looking glass. NATURE 299 (5879):103-104.

Heller, M., 1980. The Gay bowel syndrome: A common problem of homosexual patients in the emergency department. ANNALS OF EMERGENCY MEDICINE 9(9):487-493.

Hersh, E.M., Reuben, J.M., Rios, A., and Mansell, P.W.A. 1983. Elevated thymosin alpha-1 levels associated with evidence immune dysregulation in male homosexuals with a history of infectious diseases or Kaposi's sarcoma. NEW. ENG. J. MED. 308(1):45-46.

Holland, G.N., Gottlieb, M.S. et al., 1982. Ocular disorders associated with a new severe acquired cellular immunodeficiency syndrome. AMERICAN J. OF OPTHAMOLOGY 93(4):393-402.

Hospital Practice, 1982. New cases of Kaposi's sarcoma, A.I.D.S. found in heterosexual men. HOSPITAL PRACTICE 17(9):48A-48B, 48F, 48J, 48O (Sept).

Hughes, W. T., 1978. Pneumocystis pneumonia, a plague of the immunosuppresses. JOHNS HOPKINS MEDICAI JOURNAL 143:184-192.

Hymes, K.B. et al. 1981. Kaposi's sarcoma in homosexual men—a report of eight cases. LANCET II (8247):598-600 Sept. 19.

Ito, James, Comess, K.A., Alexander, R., 1982. Pneumonia due to chlamydia trachomatis in an immunocompromised adult. NEW ENGL. J. MED. 307:(2) 95-96.

JAMA — Medical News, 1982. Acquired immunodeficiency syndrome cause(s) still elusive. JAMA Sept.

24, 1982 248(12):1423-1431.

JAMA — Medical News, 1982. Neurological complications now characterizing many A.I.D.S. victims. JAMA 248 (22): p. 2941.

JAMA — Medical News, 1983. Preventing A.I.D.S. transmission: should blood donors be screened? JAMA, Feb. 4, 1983. 249:5, pp. 567-569.

Jensen, O.M., Mouridsen, H.T., Petersen, N.S., et al., 1982. Kaposi sarcoma in homosexual men: is it a new disease? LANCET I(8297):1027.

Jessamine, A.G., Baker, M.A., Doherty, J.M., et al., 1982. Acquired immunodeficiency disease in Canada. CMA JOURNAL 127:1161 (Dec. 15).

Johnson, Richard, Horowitz, S.N. and Frost, P., 1982. Disseminated Kaposi's sarcoma in a homosexual man. JAMA 247(12):1739-1741.

Jones, P., Proctor, S., Dickinson, A., George, S., 1983. Altered immunology in haemophilia. LANCET January 15, 1983, pp. 120-121.

Jorgensen, K.A., and Lawesson, S., 1982. Amyl nitrite and Kaposi's sarcoma in Homosexual men. NEW ENGLAND J. MED. 307(14):893-894.

Judson, F.N., Penley, K.A., Robinson, M.E., Smith, J.K. 1980. Comparative prevalence and rates of sexually transmitted diseases in heterosexual and homosexual men. AM. J. EPIDEMIOLO. 112: 836-843.

Katongole-Mbidde, E.K., 1982. Management of Kaposi's sarcoma. [Editorial reply] LANCET II (8297):563; Sept. 4.

Kazal, H.L., Sohn, N., Carrasco, J.I., et al., 1976. The gay bowel syndrome: clinico-pathologic correlation in 260 cases. ANN CLIN. LAB. SCI. 1976(6):184-192.

Kornfeld, H., et al., 1982. T-lymphocyte subpopulations in homosexual men. NEW ENGL. J. MED. 307(12):729-731.

Koziner, B., Denney, T., Myskowski, P., et al., 1982 Opportunistic infections and Kaposi's sarcoma in homosexual men. NEW ENGL. J. MED. 306:933.

Kwok, Shiu, O'Donnell, J., and Wood, I., 1982. Retinal cotton wool spots in a patient with pneumocystis carinii infection. NEW ENGL. J. MED. 306:184-185.

Lancet (Editorial) 1981. Sexual transmission of enteric pathogens. LANCET II(8259):1328-1329 (Dec. 12).

Laurens, R.G., Pine, J.R., Schwarzmann, S.W., 1982. PNEUMOCYSTIS CARINII pneumonia in a male homosexual. SOUTHER MED. J. 75(5):638-639 (May).

Leach, R.D., Ellis, H., 1981. Carcinoma of the rectum in male homosexuals. J. OF THE ROYAL SOCIETY OF MEDICINE 74(7):490-491 (July).

Lederman, M.M., Ratnoff, O.D., Scillain, J.J., et al., 1983. Impaired cell-mediated immunity in patients with classic hemophilia. NEW ENGL. J. MED. 308(2):79-83.

Levine, A.S., 1982. The epidemic of acquired immune dysfunction in homosexual men and its sequelae —opportunistic infections, Kaposi's sarcoma, and other malignancies: an update and interpretation. CANCER TREATMENTS REPORTS 66(6):1391-1395.

Liautaud, B., Laroche, C., Duvivier, J. et al., 1982. Le sarcome de Kaposi (maladie de Kaposi) est-il frequent en Haiti? 18th Congress des Medecins Francophones de l'Hemisphere Americain, April 1982, Port au Prince, Haiti.

Mansell, Peter W. 1982. Kaposi's sarcoma—an emerging epidemic. THE CANCER BULLETIN 34(3): 72-74.

Marmor, M., Laubenstein, L., William D., et al., 1982. Risk factors for Kaposi's sarcoma in homosexual men. LANCET I(8281):1083-1087; May 15.

Marx, J.L. 1982. New disease baffles medical community. SCIENCE 217(4560):618-621.

Masci, J.R., Nichols, P., 1983. Precautions recommended in treating patients with A.I.D.S. NEW ENG-
LAND J. MED. 308(3):156.

Masur, H., Michelis, M.A., Greene, J.B., et al., 1981. An outbreak of community acquired PNEUMO-
CYSTIS CARINII pneumonia. NEW ENGL. J. MED. 305 1431-1438.

Maurice, P., Smith, N., and Pinching, A., 1982. Kaposi's sarcoma with benign course in a homosexual.
LANCET 1982i:412-415.

McMillan, A., et al., 1981. Sigmoidoscopic and microscopic appearance of the rectal mucosa in homosexual men. GUT 22(12):1-35-1041 (Dec.)

McTighe, A.H., 1982. Association of Kaposi's sarcoma and opportunistic infections in homosexuals.
LAB MED. 13(10):633-636 (Oct).

Medical World News, 1982. Hunt steps up for cause of deadly syndrome on the rise among gay men.
MWR 23(8):19 (April 12).

Medical World News, 1982. [A.I.D.S. review]. MEDICAL WORLD NEWS, Aug. 16, pp. 7-9.

Medical World News, 1983. New evidence suggests A.I.D.S. is transmitted in donor blood. MWR January
10, pp. 8-10.

Menitove, J.E., Aster, R., et al., 1983. T-lymphocyte subpopulations in patients with classic hemophilia
treated with cryoprecipitate and lyophilized concentrates. NEW ENGL. J. MED. 308(2):83-86.

Mildvan, Donna, Gelb, A., et al., 1977. Veneral transmission of enteric pathogens in male homosexuals.
JAMA 238(13):1387-1389 (Sept. 26).

Mildvan, Donna, Mathur, U., Enlow, R., et al., 1982. Opportunistic infections and immune deficiency
in homosexual men. ANNALS OF INTERNAL MED. 96(pt. 1):700-704.

Miller, J.R., Barrett, R., Britton, C., B., et al. 1982. Progressive Multifocal Leukoencephalopathy in a
male homosexual with T-cell immune deficiency. THE NEW ENGL. J. MEDICINE 307:1436-
1438; Dec. 2.

Morriss, L., Distenfeld, A., Amorosi, E., Karpatkin, S., 1982. Autoimmune thrombocytopenic purpura in
homosexual men. ANN. INT. MED. 96(pt 1):714-717.

Morris, L. B., et al., 1982. Increased apparent autoimmune thrombocytopenic purpura (ATP) in homosexual men. CLINICAL RESEARCH 30(2):A324.

Myskowski, P. L., Romano, J. F., Safai, B., 1982. Kaposi's sarcoma in young homosexual men. CUTIS
39(1):31-34 (Jan).

Nahas, Gabriel, G., 1982. Opportunistic infections and Kaposi's sarcoma in homosexual men. NEW
ENGL. J. MED. 306-932; April 15.

Navarro, Carlos, and Hagstrom, J., 1982. Opportunistic infections and Kaposi's sarcoma in homosexual
men. NEW ENGL. J. MED. April 15, 1982:933.

Navin, H., 1981. Medical and surgical risks in handballing: implications of an inadequate socialization
process. JOURNAL OF HOMOSEXUALITY 6(3):67-76.

Neumann, H.H. 1982. Use of steroid creams as a possible cause of immunosuppression in homosexual
men. NEW ENGL. J. MED. 306:934-935; April 15.

New England J. Medicine. 1982. Special report. Epidemiological Aspects of the current outbreak of
Kaposi's sarcoma and opportunistic infections. NEW ENGL. J. MED. 306:248-252.

Nichols, P. W., 1982. Opportunistic infections and Kaposi's sarcoma in homosexual men. NEW ENGL.
J. MED. 306:934:935; April 15.

Ohara, N., Chang, S., et al., 1982. Kaposi's sarcoma and the HLA-DR5 alloantigen. ANNALS OF INT.

MED. 97(4):617 (Oct).

Oswald, G. et al., 1982. Attempted immune stimulation in the "Gay Compromise Syndrome." BRIT. MED. J. 285:1082.

Pennington, J.E., 1982. Pneumonia in the immunocompromised patient. J. OF RESP. DISEASES, 3(12): 25 (Dec.).

Phillips, S. C., et al., 1981. Sexual transmission of enteric protozoa and helminths in a venereal disease clinic population. NEW ENGL. J. MED. 305(11):603-606.

Quinn, Thomas, Corey, L., et al., 1981. The etiology of anorectal infections in homosexual men. AMERICAN J. MEDICINE 71(3):395-406 (Sept).

Quinn, Thomas, C., Goodell, Steven, E., Mkrtichian, P. A., et al., 1981. CHLAMYDIA TRACHOMATIS proctitis. [in homosexual men] NEW ENGL. J. MED. 305:195-200.

Ragni, M.V., Lewis, J. H., Spero, J. A., Bontempo, F. A., 1983. Acquired-immunodeficiency-like syndrome in two haemophiliacs. LANCET January 29, p. 213.

Reiner, N. E., Judson, F. N., Bond, W., et al., 1982. Asymptomatic rectal mucosal lesions and hepatitis B surface antigen at sites of sexual contact in homosexual men with persistent hepatitis B virus infection: evidence for de-facto parenteral transmission. ANNALS OF INTERNAL MED. 96(2): 170-173 (Feb).

Reuben, J.M., Hersh, E.M., Mansell, P. W., Newell, G., et al., 1983. Immunological characterization of homosexual males. CANCER RESEARCH 43:897-904; Feb.

Robertson, D.H. et al., 1982. Sexual Transmission of enteric pathogens. LANCET 1 (8268):393 (Feb. 13).

Rosenbaum, W., et al., 1982. Multiple opportunistic infections in a male homosexual in France. LANCET 1(8271):572-573.

Rosenfelt, F. P., et al., 1983. Non-hodgkin's lymphoma in homosexual men. WESTERN J. MED. 138(1): (January).

Rutsaert, J., Melot, C., et al., 1980. Complications infectieuses pulmonaries et neurologigues d'un sarcome de Kaposi. ANNALES D.ANATOMIE PATHOLOGIGUE 25:125-138.

Ryning, F. W., Mills, J. 1979. PNEUMOCYSTIS CARINII, TOXOPLASMA GONDII, cytomegalovirus and the compromised host. WESTERN J. MED. 130:18-34.

Schmerin, M.J., Gelston, A., Jones, T. C., 1977. Amebiasis: an increasing problem among homosexuals in New York City. JAMA 238(13):1386-1387.

Schreeder, M. T., Thompson, S. E., Hadler, S. C., et al., 1982. Hepatitis B in Homosexual men: prevalence of infection and factors related to transmission. J. OF INFECTIOUS DISEASES 146(1):7-15.

Scully, R. E., Mark, E. J., et al., 1982. Case records of the Massachusetts General Hospital: a 29-yr. old man with cryoglobulinemia, glomerulonephritis and lymphadenopathy. NEW ENGL. J. MED. 306(11):657-668.

Siegal, Frederick P., et al. 1981. Severe acquired immunodeficiency in male homosexuals, manifested by chronic perianal ulcerative herpes simplex lesions. THE NEW ENGL. J. MED. 305:1439-1444.

Singer, C. Armstrong, D., et al., 1975. PNEUMOCYSTIS CARINII pneumonia: a cluster of eleven cases. ANNALS OF INTERNAL MED. 82:772-777.

Smith, L. H., Golden, J., 1982. Medical staff conference University of California San Francisco: Pneumocystis lung disease in homosexual men. THE WESTERN J. MED. 137(5):400-407.

Snider, W. D., Simpson, D. M., et al., 1983. Primary lymphoma of the nervous system associated with acquired immune deficiency syndrome. NEW ENGL. J. MED. 308(1):45 (Jan 6).

Spiers A. and Robbins, C., 1982. Cytomegalovirus infection simulating lymphoma in a homosexual man.

LANCET I(8283):1248-1349; May 19.

Stahl, R., Friedman-Kien, A. E., Dubin, R., et al., 1982. Immunologic abnormalities in homosexual men: relationship to Kaposi's sarcoma. AM.J. MED. 73:171-177.

Thomsen, H.K., et al., 1981. Kaposi's sarcoma among homosexual men in Europe. LANCET II(8248): 688 (Sept. 26).

Ulbright, Thomas M., and Santa Cruz, Daniel J., 1981. Kaposi's Sarcoma: Relationship with hematologic, lymphoid and thymus neoplasia. CANCER 47:963-973.

U.S. House of Representatives 1982. Kaposi's Sarcoma and related opportunistic infections: Hearing before the Subcommittee on Health and the Environment. Serial No. 97-125. U.S. Gov't Printing Office.

Urban Health, 1982. A.I.D.S.: An u-date, URBAN HEALTH, August, p. 33, et seq.

Vanley, G., et al., 1982. Atypical PNEUMOCYSTIS CARINII pneumonia in homosexual men with unusual immunodeficiency. AMERI. J. ROENTGENOLOGY 138(6):1037-1041 (June).

Vaisrub, S. 1982. Homosexuality: A risk factor in infectious disease. JAMA 348(13):1402 (Sept. 26).

Vieira, J., Frank, E. et al., 1982. Acquired Immune Deficiency in Haitians — Opportunistic Infections in previously healthy Haitian immigrants. NEW ENGL. J. MED. 308(3):125-129.

Vilaseca, J., Arnau, J. M., et al., 1982. Kaposi's sarcoma and TOXOPLASMA GONDII brain abscess in a Spanish homosexual. LANCET I(8271):572 (March 6).

Waldhorn, Richard E., Tsou, E., and Kerwin, D.M., 1982. PNEUMOCYSTIS CARINII pneumonia in a previously healthy adult. JAMA 247(13):1860-1861.

Wallace, J., Coral, F., Rimm, I., et al., 1982. T-cell ratios in homosexuals. LANCET I(8277):908; April 17.

Wallace, Joyce, I., Downes, J., et al., 1983. T-Cell ratios in New York City prostitutes. LANCET I (8314 /5):58; Jan. 1/8.

William, D. C. Shookhoff, H.B., Felman, Y.M., et al., 1978. High rates of enteric protozoal infection in selected homosexual men attending a venereal disease clinic. SEX TRANSM. DIS. 1978(5):155-157.

Williams, G., Stretton, T. B., 1960. Cytomegalic inclusion disease and PNEUMOCYSTIS CARINII infection in an adult. LANCET II:951-955.

Wood, Ronald W. 1982. Opportunistic infections and Kaposi's sarcoma in homosexual men. NEW ENGL. J. MED. 306:932; April 15.

Ziegler, J. L., Miner, R. C., Rosenbaum, E., et al., 1982. Outbreak of Burkitt's-like lymphoma in homosexual men. LANCET II(8299):631-632 Sept. 18.

Immunosuppression and Pathogenesis of A.I.D.S. and Associated Diseases including "Classic" Kaposi Sarcoma; HLA Types Subsection: Parsitism and Immune Suppression

Armstong, J. A., Evans, A. S., Rao, N., Ho, M. 1976. Viral infections in renal transplant recipients. INFECTIOUS IMMUNOL. 14:970-975.

Battisto, J. R. and Chase, M. W., 1965. Induced unresponsibeness to simple allergenic chemicals. II. Independence of delayed-type hypersensitivity and the formation of circulating antibody. J. EXP. MED. 121:591-606.

Costa, Jose, and Rabson, Alan S., 1983. Generalized Kaposi's sarcoma is not a neoplasm. LANCET I(8314 /5):58 Jan 1/8.

Cunningham-Rundles, C., Cunningham-Rundles, S., Iwata, T. et al., 1981. Zinc deficiency, depressed tymic hormones and T-lymphocyte dysfunction in patients with hypogammaglobulinemia. CLIN.

IMMUNO. AND IMMUNOPATH. 21:387-396.

Cursons, R., Brown, T., Keys, E., et al., 1980. Immunity to pathogenic free-living amoebae: role of humoral antibody. INFECTION AND IMMUNITY 29(2):401-407.

Dantzig, Paul, I. 1974. Kaposi sarcoma and Polymyositis. ARCH. DERMATOL. 110:605.

Dent, P. B. 1972. Immunodepression by oncogenic viruses. PROG. MED. VIROL 14:1-35.

Dobozy, A., Husz, S., Hunyadi, J., et al., 1973. Immune deficiencies and Kaposi's sarcoma. LANCET II: 625.

Doubloug, J. H., Forre, O., Chattopadhyay, C., and Natvig, J. B., 1982. Concanavalin A induces suppressor cell activity in both T-gamma and T-non gamma cells: Most of the suppressor cells do not carry HLA-DR antigens. SCAND. J. IMMUNOL. 15:87-95.

Doyle, T. J., Venkatachalam, K. K., Maeda, K., et al., 1983. Hodgkin's Disease in renal transplant recipients. CANCER 51:245 (Jan. 15).

Dunk, A., Jenkins, W. J. and S. Sherlock. 1982. Guillain-Barre syndrome associated with hepatitis A in a male homosexual. BR. J. VENER. DIS. 58:269-270.

Eddleston, A. L. W. F., Mondelli, M., Miele-Vergani, G., et al., 1982. Lymphocyte cytotoxicity to autologous hepatocytes in chronic hepatitis B virus infection. HEPATOLOGY 2(2):122(S)-127(S).

Epstein, E. 1972. Letter: Kaposi's sarcoma and parapsoraisis en plaque in brothers. JAMA 219:1477-1478.

Fagiolo, E. 1982 Thymocytotoxic antibodies in patients with autoimmune hemolytic anemia systemic lupus erythematosus and lymphoproliferative diseases BLUT 44:225-230.

Fauci, Anthony S., et al. 1980. Drug-induced T and B lymphocyte and monocyte dysfunction. In: Infections in the Abnormal Host, M. H. Grieco, New York, New York Medical Books, pp. 163-182.

Fernandes, G., Nair, M., Onoe, K. et al., 1979. Impairment of cell-mediated immunity functions by dietary zinc deficiency in mice. PNAS 76:457-461.

Festenstein, H., Halim, K., and Arnaiz-Villena, 1978. HLA antigens on human spermatozoa. In: SPERMS, ANTIBODIES AND INFERTILITY, eds: J. Cohen and W. F. Hendry, Blackwell Scientific Pubs.

Frizzera, G., Moran, E. M. Rappaport, H. 1975. Antioimmunoblastic lymphadenopathy — Diagnosis and clinical course. AMERICAN J. MED. 59:803-818 (Dec. 1975).

Gagne, R. W., and Wilson-Jones, E. 1978. Kaposi's sarcoma and immunosuppressive therapy: an appraisal. CLIN. EXP. DERMATOL. 1978 3:135-146.

Gallis, H. A., Berman, R. A., Cate, T. R., et al., 1975. Fungal infection following renal transplantation. ARCH. INTERN. MED. 135:1163-1172.

Gaston, J. S. H., Rickinson, A. B., Epstein, M. A., 1982. Epstein Barr virus specific T-cell memory in renal allograph recipients under long term immunosuppression. LANCET I (8278)24:923-925.

Goedert, J. J. 1982. Amyl nitrate may alter T lymphocytes in homosexual men. LANCET (1982(1):412-416.

Goode, E. and Troiden, R. R., 1979. Amyl nitrate use among homosexual men. THE AMERICAN J. PSYCHIATRY 136:1067-1069.

Greene, M. H., 1982. Non-hodgkin's lymphoma and mycosis fungoides. IN: Schottenfeld, M., Fraumeni, J., CANCER EPIDEMIOLOGY AND PREVENTION. Philadelphia: Saunders pp. 754-778, 1982.

Haim, S., Shafrir, A., Better, O. 1972. Kaposi's sarcoma in association with immunosuppressive therapy. ISRAEL J. OF MEDICAL SCIENCES 8:1993-1997.

Hanrahan, D. W., Frizzera, G. et al., 1982. Opportunistic infections in prisoners. NEW ENGL. J. MED. 307(8):498 (August 19).

Hanto, Douglas W. Frizzera, G., Gajl-Peczalska et al., 1982. Epstein Barr virus induced B-Cell lymphoma after renal transplantation. NEW ENGL. J. MED 306(15):913-918 (April 15).

Hardy, E., Goldbareb, M. A., Levine, S., et al., 1976. Kaposi's sarcoma in renal transplantation. CANCER 38:144.

Harwood, A. R., Osora, D., Hofstader, S. L., et al. 1979. Kaposi's sarcoma in recipients of renal transplants. AM. J. MED. 67:759-767.

Hauser, W., Luft, B. J. et al., 1982. CNS toxoplasmosis in homosexual and heterosexual adults. NEW ENGL. J. MED. 307(8):498-499 (Aug. 19).

Horne, M. K., Waterman, M. R., Simon, L. M., et al., 1979. Methemoglobinemia from sniffing butyl nitrite. ANNALS OF INT. MED. 91:417-418.

Hoshaw, R. A., Schwartz, R. A., 1980. Kaposi's sarcoma after immunosuppressive therapy with prednisone. ARCH. OF DERMATOL. 166:1280-1282.

Hughes, W. T., 1978. Pneumocystis pneumonia, a plague of the immunosuppressed. JOHNS HOPKINS MEDICAL JOURNAL 143:184-192.

Jackson, C. D., 1981. Working paper on volatile nitrites. National Center for Toxicology Program (NTP); Jefferson, Ark., 1981.

Jensen, J. R. and From, E., 1982. Alteration in T lymphocytes and T-lymphocyte subpopulations in patients with symphilis. BR. J. VEN. DISEASES 58:18-22.

Jorgensen, K. A., and Lawesson, S., 1982. Amyl nitrite and Kaposi's sarcoma in Homosexual men. NEW ENGLAND J. MED 307(14):893-894.

Judson, F. N., Penley, K. A., Robinson, M. E., Smith, J. K. 1980. Comparative prevalence and rates of sexually transmitted diseases in heterosexual and homosexual men. AM. J. EPIDEMIOLO. 112:836-843.

Kean, B. H. 1981. Clinical amebiasis in New York City: Symptoms, Sights and Treatment. BULL. NY ACAD. MED. 57:207-211.

Klepp, O., Dahl, O., Hofstader, S. L., et al., 1978. Association of Kaposi sarcoma and prior immunosuppressive therapy: a five year material of Kaposi's sarcoma in Norway. CANCER 42:2626-2630.

Klein, M. B., Pereira, F. A., and Kantor, I. 1974. Kaposi's sarcoma complicating systemic lupus erythromatosus treated with immunosuppression. ARCH. DERMATOL. 110:602-605.

Kobiler, D., and Mirelman, D., 1980. A lectin activity in entamoeba histolytica trophozoites. ARCHIVO INVEST. MED.(MEXICO) 11(Suppl. 1):101.

Krueger, G., Malmgren, R., and Berhard, C., 1971. Malignant Lymphoma and plasmacytosis in mice under prolonged immunosuppression and persistent antigenic stimulation. TRANSPLANTATION 11(2):138-144.

Kuntz, M., Innes, J. B. and Weksler, M. E. 1979. The cellular basis of the impaired autologous mixed lymphocyte reaction in patients with systemic lupus erythmatosus J. CLIN. INVESTIG. 63:151.

Lang, D. J., Kummer, J. F., Hartly, D. P., 1975. Cytomegalovirus in semen: Observations in selected populations. THE J. OF INFECTIOUS DISEASES 132:472-473.

Leung, F., Fam, A. G., Osoba, D. 1981. Kaposi's sarcoma complicating corticosteroid therapy for temporal arteritis. AM. J. MED. 71:320-322.

MacDonald, T. T., 1982. Immunosuppression caused by antigen feeding I. Incidence for the activation of a feedback suppressor pathway in the spleens of antigen-fed mice. EUR. J. IMMUNOL. 12:767-773.

Master, S. P., Taylor, J. F., Kyalwazi, S. K., and Zeigler, J. L., 1970. Immunological studies in Kaposi's sarcoma in Uganda. BR. MED. J. I:600-602.

Mattern, C., Caspar-Natovitz, D. 1980. Detection of antibodies against lectin-like "toxin" of entamoeba histolytica in sera of patients with invasive amebiasis. ARCHIVOS DE INVESTIG. MED(MEX.)

11 (Suppl. 1):143.

McDonough, R. J., Madden, J. J., Falek, A., et al., 1980. Alteration of T and null cell lymphocyte frequencies in the peripheral blood of human opiate addicts: in vivo evidence for opiate receptor sites on T lymphocytes. J. IMMUNOL. 125:2539-2543.

Meyers, J. D., Flournoy, N., and Thomas, E.D., 1980. Cytomegalovirus infection and specific cell-mediated immunity after bone marrow transplantation. J. INFEC. DISEASES 142:816-824.

Moreb, J., Okon, E., Matzner, Y., Polliack, A. 1983. Angioblastic lymphadenopathy. CANCER 51:487-491 (Feb. 1).

Ohara, N., Chang, S., et al., 1982. Kaposi's sarcoma and the HLA-DR5 alloantigen. ANNALS OF INT. MED. 97(4):617 (Oct.).

Pekarek, R., Sandstead, H., Jacob, R. et al., 1979. Abnormal cellular immune responses during acquired zinc deficiency. AM. J. CLIN. NUTR. 32:1466-1471.

Penn, I. 1979. Kaposi's sarcoma in organ transplant recipients: report of 20 cases. TRANSPLANTATION 27:8-11.

Pollack, M. S., Kirkpatrick, D. Kapoor, N. et al. 1982. Identification by HLA typing of intrauterine-derived maternal T cells in four patients with severe combined immunodeficiency. NEW ENGL. J. MED. 307(11):662-666.

Prakash, C. and Lang, R. W. 1980. Studies on immune fertility: a hypothesis on the etiology of immune infertility based on the biological role of seminal plasma immune response inhibitor. MT. SINAI J. MED. (NY) 47:491-510.

Quinnan, G. V., Manischewitz, J. E., Ennis, F. A., 1980. Role of cytotoxic T lymphocytes in murine cytomegalovirus infection. J. GEN. VIROL. 47:503-508.

Reinherz, E. L., O'Brien, C., Rosentha, P., and Schlossman, S. F., 1980. The cellular basis for viral-induced immunodeficiency: analysis by monoclonal antibodies. J. IMMUNOL. 125:1269-1274.

Rinaldo, Charles R., et al. 1980. Mechanisms of immunosuppression in cytomegalovirus mononucleosis. THE J. OF INFECTIOUS DISEASES 141(4):488-495.

Rodriguez-Cordoba, S. and Arnaiz-Villena, A., 1982. Human seminal cells other than spermatozoa stimulate lymphocyte cultures. TISSUE ANTIGENS 19:313-314.

Ryning, F. W., Mills, J. 1979. PNEUMOCYSTIS CARINII, TOXOPLASMA GONDII, cytomegalovirus and the compromised host. WESTERN J. MED. 130:18-34.

Saemunson, A. K., Albeck, H., Hansen, J. P. H., Nielsen, N. H., et al., 1982. Epstein-Barr virus in naso-pharyngeal and salivary gland carcinomas of Greenland Eskimoes. BRITISH J. CANCER 46:721-728.

Sridama, V., pacini, F., Yang, S., et al., 1982. Decreased levels of helper cells: a possible cause of immunodeficiency in pregnancy. NEW ENG. J. MED. 307:352-356 Aug. 5.

Straus, D. J., Filippa, D. A., Lieberman, P. H., Koziner, B., et al., 1983. The non-Hodgkin's lymphomas. CANCER 51:101-109 (Jan. 1).

Thomas, H. C., Brown, D., Routhier, G., et al., 1982. Inducer and Suppressor T-cells in Hepatitis B virus-induced liver disease. HEPATOLOGY 2(2):202-204.

Veltri, R. W., Shah, S. H., McClung, J. E., Clingberg, W. G., et al., 1983. Epstein-Barr virus fatal infectious monomucleosis and Hodgkin's disease in siblings. CANCER 51:509-520 (Feb. 1).

Walker, Jonathan, E., Cook, J. D., Harrison P., and Stastny, P., 1982. HLA and the Response of lymphocytes to Viral antigens in patients with multiple sclerosis. HUMAN IMMOLOGY 4:71-78.

Wallace, Joyce, I., Downes, J., et al., 1983. T-Cell ratios in New York City prostitutes. LANCET I(8314/5) :58 Jan. 1/8.

Weksler, M. E., and Kozak, R. 1977. Lymphocyte transformation induced by autologous cells V. Generation of immunlogic memory and specificity during the autologous mixed lymphocyte reaction. J. EXP. MED. 146:1833.

Wettstein, P. J. and Bailey, D. W., 1982. Immunodominance in the immune response to "multiple" histocompatibility antigens. IMMUNOGENETICS 16:47-58.

Williams, G., Stretton, T. B., 1960. Cytomegalic inclusion disease and PNEUMOCYSTIS CARINII infection in an adult. LANCET II:951-955.

Woodruff, J. F., and Woodruff, J. J. 1975. The effect of viral infections on the function of the immune system. In: Notkins, A. L., ed. VIRAL IMMUNOLOGY AND IMMUNOPATHOLOGY New York: Academic Press, 1975:393-418.

Woodruff, J. M., Hansen, J. A., Good, R. A. et al., 1976. The pathology of the graft vs. host reaction in adults receiving bone marrow transplants. TRANSPL. PROCEED. 8:675-684.

Yu, D. T. Y., Winchester, R. J., Fu, S. M., et al., 1980. Peripheral blood Ia-positive cells. Increases in certain diseases and after immunization. J. EXP. MED 151-91-100.

Parasitism and Immune Suppression

South African Medical Journal, 1982. Immunodeficiency and homosexuality. SAMJ 61(9):298.

Ament, M.E., and Rubin, C. D., 1972. Relation of giardiasis to abnormal intestinal structure and function in gastrointestinal immunodeficiency syndromes. GASTROENTEROLOGY 62:216.

Anders, R. F., et al. 1982. Giardiasis in mice: Analysis of humoral and cellular immune responses to GIARDIA MURIS. PARASITE IMMUNOLOGY 4:47-57.

Bolan, R., Owen, R. L., 1980. Are lactating mothers a source of giardiasis? NEW ENGL J. MED., 303: 820 Sept. 23.

Carswell, F., et al., 1981. Nutritional status, globulin titers and parasitic infections of two populations of Tanzanian school children. THE AM. J. CLIN. NUTR. 34:1292.

Cruickshank, J. K., and Mackensie, C. 1981. Immunodiagnosis in parasitic disease. BRIT. MED. J. 283: 1349-1350.

Davies, et al., 1980. The biological significance of the immune response with special reference to parasites and cancer. J. PARASITOLOGY 66:705.

Despommier, D. C. 1981. The laboratory diagnosis of E. HISTOLYTICA. BULL. N.Y. ACAD. MED. 57(3):212-216.

Dixon, J. B., et al., 1982. Immune recognition of ECHINOCOCCUS GRANULOSUS I. Parasite-activated primary transformation by normal murine lymph node cells. PARASITE IMMUNOL. 4(1):33-45.

Dritz, S. 1980. Medical Aspects of Homosexuality. NEW ENGL. J. MED. 302(8):463-464.

Faubert, G. M. 1982. The reversal of the immunodepression phenomenon in trichinellosis and its effect on the life cycle of the parasite. PARASITE IMMUNOLO. 4:13-20.

Fodor, T. 1981. Unanswered questions about the transmission of amediasis. BULL N.Y. ACAD. SCI. 57(3):224.

Gill, H. S. 1982. Prevalence of antibodies against parasitic infections in Tansanian Blood Donors at Dar es Salaam. THE CENT. AFRICAN J. MED. 28(2):38-40.

Gold, D. et al., 1978. Immunological studies on hamsters infected with ENTAMOEBA HISTOLYTICA. J. PARASITOLOGY 64:866.

Imperato, P. J. 1981. Conclusions about amebiasis. BULL. N.Y. ACAD MED. 57:240.

75080

Kamal, B. H. and G. I. Higashi, 1982. Suppression of mitogen-induced lymphocyte transformation by plasma from patients with hepatosplenic SCHISTOMAIASIS MANSONI: role of immune complexes. PARASITE IMMUNOLOGY 4:283.

Kazal, H. L., Sohn, N., Carrasco, J. I., et al., 1976. The gay bowel syndrome: clinico-pathologic correlation in 260 cases. ANN CLIN. LAB. SCI. 6(2):184-192.

Kean, B. H. 1981. Clinical amebiasis in New York City: symptoms, signs and treatment. BULL. N.Y. ACAD. MED. 57:207.

Keystone, J. S. 1981. Imported intestinal parasites: A growing problem? CMA JOURNAL 125:415-417.

Kobiler, D., and Mirelman, D., 1980. A lectin activity in entameba histolytica trophozoites. ARCH. INVESTIG. MED. (MEX) Suppl. 1 11:101.

Mansfield, J. M., and Wallace, J. H., 1974. Suppression of cell-mediated immunity in experimental African Trypanosomiasis. INFECT. IMMUNOL. 10:335.

McMillan, A., et al., 1981. Sigmoidoscopic and microscopic appearance of the rectal mucosa in homosexual men. GUT 22(12):1035-1041 (Dec.).

Mildvan, Donna, Gleb, A., et al., 1977. Venereal transmission of enteric pathogens in male homosexuals. JAMA 238(13):1387-1398 (Sept. 26).

Miller, C. H., Malcolm, R. M., et al., 1983. Coccidiodomycosis: Early immunologic findings. WEST. J. MED. 138(1):55.

Noble, E. R., and Noble, G. A., 1982. Parasitology: The biology of animal parasites. Lea and Febinger, Philadelphia, 1982.

Nussenzwieg, R. 1982. Parasitic disease as a cause of immune suppression. NEW ENGL. J. MED. 306-423.

Ottesen, E. A., 1979. Modulation of the host response to human schistomasis. I. Adherent suppressor cells that inhibit lymphocyte proliferative responses to parasite antigens. J. IMMUNOL. 123:1639.

Parasitic Diseases on the rise, but new drugs coming. AMERICAN PHARMACY NS21(11):13-17.

Pherson, P. O., et al. 1981. The "Gay Bowel Syndrome" and amebiasis as sexually transmitted diseases in Sweden. LAKARTIDNINGEN 78(35):2924 (Aug. 26).

Phillips, S. C., et al., 1981. Sexual transmission of enteric protozoa and helminths in a venereal disease clinic population. NEW ENGL. J. MED. 305(11):603-606.

Schmerin, M. J., Gelston, A., Jones, T. C., 1977. Amebiasis: an increasing problem among homosexuals in New York City. JAMA 238(13):1386-1387.

Sorvillo, F. and Ash, L., 1982. Parasitic diseases in Karamoja, Uganda. THE LANCET I(8277):912 April 17.

Takukama, T. Kuhner, A. L., et al., 1976. Biological expressions of lymphocyte activation V. Characterization of a soluble immune response inhibitor produced by ConA spleen cells. J. IMMUNOLO 117:323.

Ulbright, Thomas M., and Santa Cruz, Daniel J., 1981. Kaposi's Sarcoma: Relationship with hematologic, lymphoid and thymus neoplasia. CANCER 47:963-973.

Vadas, M. A., 1980. Parasite Immunity and the major Histocompatibility comples. IMMUNOGENETICS 22:215-223.

Vaisrub, S. 1982. Homosexuality: A risk factor in infectious disease. JAMA 238(13):1402 (Sept. 26).

Wellhausen, S. R., and Mansfield, J. M., 1979. Lymphocyte function in experimental African Trypanosomiasis II. Spleenic suppressor cell activity. THE J. OF IMMUNOL. 122:818.

Effects of Putative Con-A Like Lectin Produced by E. Histolytica

Bramwell, V. H. C., Crowther, D., et al., 1982. Studies of lectin binding to normal and neoplastic lymphoid tissues I. Normal Nodes and Hodgkin's disease. BRIT. J. CANCER 46:568.

Gullberg, M. and Larsson, E., 1982. Studies of induction and effector functions of Con-A induced suppressor cells that limit TCGF (T cell growth factor) production. J. OF IMMUNOL. 128(2):746.

Howard, M. et al., 1981. Quantitation of binding of Factor VIII antigen to Con A BRITISH J. HEMATOL. 47:607-615.

Kuwata, T., Fuse, A., et al., 1980. Effects of Con A on the anti-viral and cell growth inhibitory action of human interferons. ANNALS N.Y. ACAD. SCI 350:211.

Mioduszewska, O. et al., 1981. Immunosuppressive effect of Con A IV: The effect of Con A on the local graft vs. host reaction in the mouse popliteal lymph node. ARCHIVUM IMMUNOL. THER. EXP. 29:385.

Renata, M. 1980. The immunosuppressive effects of ConA III. Influence on the survival time of skin allografts in mice. ARCHIVUM. IMMUNOL. THER. EXP. 28:635.

Vitiello, A., et al., 1980. Con A induces a T-cell dependent activation of Human tonsil B cells in vitro. THYMUS 1:215-223.

Zenian, A. and Kierszenbaum, F., 1982. Inhibition of macrophage-TRYPANOSOMA CRUZI interaction by concanavalin A and differential binding of bloodstream and culture forms to the macrophage surface. J. PARISITOL. 68(3):408-415.

Therapeutic Modalities (see also Idiopathic Thrombocytopenic Purpura)

Avrin, A. M., Yeager, S. A., Merigan, T. C., 1976. Effect of leukocyte interferon on urinary excretion of cytomegalovirus by infants. J. INFECTIOUS DIS. 133:A205-210.

Bach, J., Bach, M., Charreire and Le Brauchau, Y., 1980. Thymic hormones and immune regulation. In: IMMUNOREGULATION AND AUTOIMMUNITY Eds: Krakauer and Cathcart. Elsevier North Holland, Inc. 1980.

Balfour, H. H., Bean, B., Mitchell, C. D., et al. 1982. Acyclovir in immunocompromised patients with cytomegalovirus disease. A controlled trial at one institution. THE AMERICAN JOURNAL OF MEDICINE—ACYCLOVIR SYMPOSIUM Summer supplement:pp. 241-248.

Bissell, M. J., Hatie, C., Farson, D., et al., 1980 Ascorbic acid inhibits replication and infectivity of avian RNA tumor virus. PNAS 77(5):2711-2715.

Broder, Samuel, Muul, L., and Waldeman. 1978. Suppressor cells in neoplastic disease. J. NAT. CANCER SOC. 61:5-11.

Bryk, D., Farman, J., Dallenmand, S. et al., 1978. Kaposi's sarcoma of the gastrointestinal tract: roentgen manifestations. GASTROINTEST. RADIO. 3:425-430.

Cheesman, S. H., Rubin, R. H., Stewart, J. A., et al., 1979 Controlled clinical trial of prophylactic human-leukocyte interferon in renal transplantation: effects on cytomegalovirus and herpes simplex virus infections. NEW ENGL. J. MED. 300(24):1345-1349.

Collins, M., and Hellmann, K. 1982. Histamine receptor antagonism and anti-tumor activity. BRITISH J. CANCER 46:817-820.

Fefer, Alexander 1979. Immunotherapy of cancer. NATIONAL CANCER INSTITUTE MONOGRAPH NO. 52, pp. 445-450.

Fefer, Alexander, Cheever, M. A., Thomas, D., et al., 1981. Bone marrow transplanatation for refractory acute leukemia in 34 patients with identical twins. BLOOD 57(3):421-429.

Fernandes, G., Nair, M., Onoe, K. et al., 1979. Impairment of cell-mediated immunity functions by dietary zinc deficiency in mice. PNAS 76:457-461.

Gabizon, A. and Trainin, N. 1980. Regulatory action of THF on T cell reactivity to mitogens. THYMUS 1:225-239.

Gange, R. W. and Jones, E. W., 1978. Kaposi's sarcoma and immunosuppressive therapy: an appraisal. CLINICAL AND EXPERIMENTAL DERMATOLOGY 3:135-146.

Gershon, R. K., Eardley, D., Durum, D., et al., 1981. Contrasuppression: A novel immunoregulatory activity. J. EXP. MED. 153:1533-1546.

Giraldo, G., Beth, E., and Kyalwazi, S. K. 1981. Etiological implications of Karposi's Sarcoma. In ANTIBIOTICS AND CHEMOTHERAPY (Schoenfeld et al., eds.), Basel, Switzerland, S. Karger, vol. 29. pp. 12-29.

Gunby, P. 1982. T-cell stimulator undergoes diverse testing.(Medical News) in JAMA 248(7):807.

Hersh, E. M., Gutterman, J. U., Mavligit, G., et al., 1973. Host defense, chemical immunosuppression and the transplant recipient. Relative effects of intermittant versus continuous immunosuppressive therapy with reference to the objectives on treatment. TRANSPLANT. PROC. 5:1191-1195.

JAMA--Medical News, 1982. Cytomegalovirus vaccine work progressing. JAMA Sept. 24, 1982 248(12): 1424-1425.

Jensen, O.M., Mouridsen, H. T., Petersen, N. S., et al., 1982. Kaposi sarcoma in homosexual men: is it a new disease? LANCET I (8279):1027.

Katongole-Mbidde, E. K., 1982. Management of Kaposi's sarcoma. [Editorial reply] LANCET II(8297): 563 Sept. 4.

Knock, F., Gascoyne, R., Sylvester, R., and Wibel, R., 1981. Ascorbic acid as a thiolprive: Ability to induce immunity against some cancers in mice. PHYSIOL. CHEM. AND PHYSICS 13:325-333.

Knodell, R., Tate, M., Akl, B., and Wilson, J. 1981. Vitamin C prophylaxis for post-transfusion hepatitis: lack of effect in a controlled trail. AM. J. CLIN. NUT. 34:20-23.

Lancet. 1979. Ascorbic acid: Immunological effects and hazards. LANCET I(8111):308.

Lang, D. J., and Cheung, K., 1982. Effectiveness of acycloguanosine and trifluorothymidine as inhibitors of cytomegalovirus infection in vitro. AMERICAN J. MED.: ACYCLOVIR SYMPOSIUM Summer 1982:49-53.

Linker, C. 1983. Plasmapheresis in clinical medicine. (Medical Progress). THE WESTERN J. MEDICINE 138(1):60-68.

Mar, E., Patel, P. C., Huang, E., 1982. Effect of [acyclovir] on viral-specific polypeptide synthesis in human cytomegalovirus-infected cells. THE AMERICAN J. MED. Acyclovir Symposium: Summer 1982:82-85.

Marder, V. J., Nusbacher, J., and Anderson, F. W. 1981. One-year follow-up of Plasma Exchange therapy in 14 patients with idiopathic thrombocytopenic purpura. TRANSFUSION 21(3):291-298.

Nicklin, S. and Shand, F., 1982. Abrogation of suppressor cell function by inhibitors of prostaglandin synthesis. INT. J. IMMUNOPHARM. 4(5):407-414.

Oliveny, C. L. M., Toya, T., Mbiddle, K. E., et al., 1974. Treatment of Kaposi sarcoma with combination of actinomycin D, vincristine, and imidazole carboxamide (NSC-45388): results of randomized clinical trials. INT. J. CANCER 14:649-656.

Oswald, G. et al., 1982. Attempted immune stimulation in the "Gay Compromise Syndrome." BRIT. MED. J. 285:1082.

Pekarek, R., Sandstead, H., Jacob, R. et al., 1979. Abnormal cellular immune responses during acquired zinc deficiency. AM. J. CLIN. NUTR. 32:1466-1471.

Plotkin, S. A., Starr, S. E., and Bryan, C. K., 1982. In vitro and In vivo responses of cytomegalovirus to acyclovir. In: ACYCLOVIR SYMPOSIUM, The American J. Medicine:257-261 (Summer 1982).

Poydock, M. E., Reikert, D., Aleandri, L., 1982. Inhibiting effect of dehydroascorbic acid on cell division in ascites tumors in mice. EXPL. CELL BIOL. 50:34-38.

Quinnan, Gerald V., Kirmani, N., Rook, A. H., et al. 1982. Cytotoxic T cells in cytomegalovirus infection: HLA-restricted T-lymphocyte and non-T-lymphocyte cytotoxic responses correlate with recovery from cytomegalovirus infection in bone-marrow-transplant recipients. NEW ENGL. J. MED. 307: 7-13.

Serrou, B., and Cupissol, D., 1981. Nutritional support and the immune system in cancer management: a critical review. CANCER TREATMENT REPORTS 65 (Suppl. 5):115-120.

Siegel, B. V., 1975. Enhancement of interferon production by poly(rI)-poly(rC) in mouse cell cultures by ascorbic acid. NATURE 254:531-532.

Siegel, J. N., Schwartz, A., et al., 1982. T-cell suppression and contrasuppression induced by histamine H-2 and H-1 receptor agonists, respectively. PNAS 79:5052-5056 (Aug).

Storb, Rainer 1982. What role for autologous marrow transplantation in cancer therapy? NATURE 295-555.

Ramirez, I., Richie, E., Wang, Y., Van Eys, J., 1980. Effect of ascorbic in vitro on lymphocyte reactivity to mitogens. J. OF NUTRITION 110:2207-2215.

Trainin, N., Small, M., Handzel, Z., and Varsand, I. 1980. Possible role of thymic hormones in the control of autoimmune processes. IN: IMMUNOREGULATION AND AUTOIMMUNITY Eds: Kralauer and Cathcart, Elsevier North Holland, 1980.

Van der Spuy, S., Levy, D. W., and Levin, W., 1980. Cimetidine in the treatment of herpesvirus infections. S. AFR. MED. J. 58(3)112-116.

Verrier, Jones J., Cumming, R. H., Bucknall, R., et al. 1976. Plasmapheresis in the management of acute sysemic lupus erythematosis. LANCET 1:709.

Winston, D. J., Lau, W. K., Gale, R. P., et al., 1980 Trimethoprimsulfamethoxazole for the treatment of PNEUMOCYSTIS CARINII pneumonia. ANN. INTERN MED. 92:762-769.

Clinical Tests and Evaluation of Immunocompetence

Centers for Disease Control, 1978. Quantitation and Functional Assay of T and B cells. Atlanta, GA: CDC Control, 1978 (Immunology Series No. 8).

Hersh, E. M., Reuben, J. M., Rios, A., and Mansell, P.W.A. 1983. Elevated thymosin alpha-1 levels associated with evidence immune dysregulation in male homosexuals with a history of infectious diseases or Kaposi's sarcoma. NEW ENG. J. MED. 308(1):45-46.

Hymes, K.B., Shulman, S., et al., 1979. A solid-phase radioimmunoassay for bound anti-platelet antibody: studies on 45 patients with autoimmune platelet disorders. JOURNAL OF LABORATORY AND CLINICAL MEDICINE 94:639-648.

England, Albert, C., Miller, S., and Maki, D., 1982. Occular findings of accute cytomegalovirus infection in an immunologically competent adult. NEW ENGL. J. MED 307-94-95 July 8.

Kornfield, H., et al., 1982. T-lymphocyte subpopulations in homosexual men. NEW ENGL. J. MED. 307(12):729-731.

Kwok, Shiu, O'Donnell, J., and Wood, I., 1982. Retinal cotton wool spots in a patient with pneumocystis carinii infection. NEW ENGL. J. MED. 306:184-185 July 15.

Lennette, E. H., Schmidt, N. J., (Eds), 1979. DIAGNOSTIC PROCEDURES FOR VIRAL, RICKETT-SIAL AND CHLAMYDIAL INFECTIONS, 5th Ed. Washington, D.C.: American Public Health Association, pp. 241-247, 327-336.

Mingnari, Maria C., Melioli, G., et al., 1982. Surface markers of cloned human T cells with helper or suppressor activity on pokeweek mitogen-driven B cell differentiation. LANCET II (8313):1431-1433.

Reuben, J. M., Hersh, E. M., Mansell, P. W., Newell, G., et al., 1983. Immunological characterization of homosexual males. CANCER RESEARCH 43:897-904; Feb.

Siegal, F. P., 1982. Normal delayed-type skin reactions in early stages of acquired cellular immunodeficiency. NEW ENGL. J. MED. 307:184 July 15.

Stagno, S., Pass, R. F., Reynolds, D. W. et al., 1980. Comparative study of diagnostic procedures for congenital cytomegalovirus infection. PEDIATRICS 65:251-7.

Stahl, R., Friedman-Kien, A. E., Dubin, R., et al., 1982. Immune abnormalities in homosexual men with Kaposi's sarcoma: relationship to Kaposi's sarcoma, AM. J. MED. 73:171-177.

Clinical Course

Anderson, B. C., 1983. Cryptosporidiosis. LAB MEDICINE 14(1)50-56.

Auerbach, D. M., Bennet, J. V., Brachman, P. S. et al., 1982. Epidemiological aspects of the current outbreak of Kaposi's sarcoma and opportunistic infections. NEW ENG. J. MED. 306:248-252.

Bart, R. S., et al., 1982. Tumor conference 41: Spontaneously disappearing Kaposi's sarcoma. JOURNAL OF DERMATOLOGIC SURGERY AND ONCOLOGY 8(4):257-259.

Brunning, R. D., Foley, J. F., Fortuny, I. E., 1963. Hodgkins disease and Kaposi's sarcoma ARCH. INTER. MED. 112:363-369.

Bryk, D., Farman, J., Dallenmand, S. et al., 1978. Kaposi's sarcoma of the gastrointestinal tract: roentgen manifestations. GASTROINTEST. RADIOL. 3:425-430.

Burke, B. A., Good, R. A., 1973. PNEUMOCYSTIS CARINII infection. MEDICINE 52:23-51.

Centers for Disease Control 1982. Diffuse, undifferentiated non-Hodgkins lymphoma among homosexual males — United States. MMWR 31(21):277-284.

———— 1982. Persistent, generalized, lymphadenopathy among homosexual males. MMWR 31(19): 249-251.

———— 1982. Cryptosporidiosis: Assessment of chemotherapy of males with A.I.D.S. MMWR 31(44): 589-591.

Durack, David J., 1981. Opportunistic infections and Kaposi's sarcoma in homosexual men. NEW ENGL. J. MED. 305:1465-1467.

Ettinger, D. S., Humphrey, R. L., and Skinner, M. D. 1975. Kaposi's sarcoma associated with multiple myeloma. JOHNS HOPKINS MED. J. 137:88-90.

Epstein, D. M. Gefter, W. B. et al., 1982. Lung disease in homosexual men. RADIOLOGY 143(1):7-10.

Friedman, A., Freeman, W., Orellana, J., et al., 1982. Cytomegalovirus retinitis and immunodeficiency in homosexual males. LANCET I (8278):958 April 24.

Gilkey, F. W., 1982. Opportunistic infections and Kaposi's sarcoma in homosexual men. NEW ENGL. J. MED. 306:933 April 15.

Giron, J. A., et al., 1982. Should inpatients with PNEUMOCYSTIS CARINII be isolated? LANCET II (8288):46 July 3.

Hanno, R., Owen, L. G., Callen, J. P., 1979. Kaposi's sarcoma with extensive silent internal involvement. INT. J. DERM. 18:718-721.

Ito, J., et al., 1982. Pneumonia due to chlamydia trachomatis in an immunocompromised adult. NEW ENG. J. MED 307 (2):95-96.

JAMA Medical News 1982. Acquired immunodeficiency syndrome cause(s) still elusive. JAMA 248(12): 1423-1431 (Sept. 24).

Jensen, O.M., et al., 1982. Kaposi's sarcoma in homosexual men: is it a new disease? LANCET I (8279): 1027.

Katongole-Mbiddle, E.K., 1982. Management of Kaposi's sarcoma. [editorial reply] LANCET II(8297): 563 Sept. 4.

Kornfeld, H., et al., 1982. T-lymphocyte subpopulations in homosexual men. NEW ENGL. J. MED. 307(12):729-731.

Kwok, Shiu, O'Donnel, et al, 1982. Retinal Cotton Wool spots in a patient with PNEUMOCYSTIS CARINII infection. NEW ENGL. J. MED. 306:184-185.

Laurens, R. G., Pine, J. R., Schwarzmann, S. W., 1982. PNEUMOCYSTIS CARINII pneumonia in a male homosexual. SOUTHER MED. J. 75(5):638-639 (May).

Levine, A. S., 1982. The epidemic of acquired immune dysfunction in homosexual men and its sequelae —opportunistic infections, Kaposi's sarcoma and other malignacies: an update and interpretation. CANCER TREATMENTS REPORTS 66(6):1391-1395.

Maurice, P. Smith, N., et al., 1982. Kaposi's sarcoma with a benign course in a homosexual. LANCET 1982:412-415 Aug. 22.

Miller, J. R., Barrett, R., et al., 1982. Progressive multifocal leukoencephalopathy in a male homosexual with T-cell immune deficiency. NEW ENGL. J. MED. 307-1436-1438. Dec. 2.

Morris, L. B., et al., 1982. Increased apparent autoimmune thrombocytopenic purpura (ATP) in homosexual men. CLINICAL RESEARCH 30(2):A324.

Reynolds, W. A., Winkelmann, R. K., and Soule, E.L.L., 1964. Kaposi's sarcoma: A clinicapathologic study with particular reference to its relationship to the reticuloendothelia system. MEDICINE 44:419.

Ryning, F. W., Mills, Jr. 1979. PNEUMOCYSTIS CARINII, TOXOPLASMA GONDII, cytomegalovirus and the compromised host. WESTERN J. MED 130:18-34.

Safai, B. and R. A. Good, 1981. Kaposi's sarcoma: A review and recent developments. CA 31:1-12.

Siegal, F. P., et al., 1981. Severe acquired immunodeficiency in male homosexuals, manifested by chronic perianal ulcerative herpes simplex lesions. NEW ENGL. J. MED. 305:1439-1444.

Smith, L. H., Golden, J., 1982. Medical staff conference University of California San Francisco: Pneumocystis lung disease in homosexual men. THE WESTERN J. MED. 137(5):400-407.

Spiers, A., and Robbins, C. 1982. Cytomegalovirus infection simulating lymphoma in a homosexual man. LANCET May 29:1248-1249.

Templeton, A.C. 1981. Kaposi's sarcoma (with 77 references). PATHOLOGY ANNUAL 16(2):315-336.

Walther, R. R. et al., 1979. TINEA PEDIS masking a Kaposi's sarcoma. INT. J. OF DERMATOLOGY 18(9):751-752 (Nove.).

Watanabe, J. M. Chinchinian, H., Weigz, C. et al., 1969. PNEUMOCYSTIS CARINII pneumonia in a family. JAMA 193:685-686.

Williams, G., Stretton, T. B., 1960. Cytomegalic inclusion disease and PNEUMOCYSTIS CARINII infection in an adult. LANCET II:951-955.

Zeigler, J. L., Miner, R. C., et al., 1982. Outbreak of Burkitt's like lymphoma in homosexual men. LAN-CET II(8299):631-632.

Cytomegalovirus, Epstien Barr, and Other Viruses Including Possible Retrovirus

Albrecht, and Rapp, F., 1973. Malignant transformation of hamster embryo fibroblasts following exposure to ultraviolet-irradiated human cytomegalovirus. VIROLOGY 55:53-61.

Betts, R. F., Freeman, R. B., Douglas, R. G., et al., 1975. Transmission of cytomegalovirus with renal allograph. KIDNEY INT. 8:385-392.

Bancroft, G. J., Shellman, G. R., and Chalmaer, J. E., 1981. Genetic influences on the augmentation of natural killer cell (NK) during murine cytomegalovirus infection: correlation with patterns of resistance. J. IMMUNO. 126:988-994.

Centers for Disease Control, 1982. Hepatitis B virus Vaccine Safety: Report of an Inter-Agency Group. MMWR 31(34):465-467.

Drew, W. L., Miner, R., Ziegler, J., et al., 1982 Cytomegalovirus and Kaposi's sarcoma in young homosexual men. LANCET II(8290):125-127.

Drew, L. W., et al. 1981. Prevalence of Cytomegalovirus infections in Homosexual men. THE J. OF INFECTIOUS DISEASES 143:188-192.

Dunk, A., Jenkins, W. J. and S. Sherlock. 1982. Guillain-Barre syndrome associated with hepatitis A in a male homosexual. BR. J. VENER. DIS. 58:269-270.

Friedman, A., Freeman, W., Orellana, J., et al., 1982. Cytomegalovirus retinitis and immunodeficiency in homosexual males. LANCET I(8278):958. April 24.

Gallo, R. C., and Wong-Staal, F., 1982. Retroviruses as etiological agents of some animal and human leukemias and lymphomas and as tools for elucidating the molecular mechanism of leukomogenesis. BLOOD 60(3):545-557.

Gartner, L., Wilhelm, J. A., and Czieschnek, 1982. In vitro stimulation of lymphocytes by different strains of Cytomegalovirus. MED. MICROBIOL. IMMUNOL. 171:53-57.

Geder, L., Lausch, R. N., O'Neill, F. J., and Rapp, F., 1976. Oncogenic transformation of human embryo lung cells by human cytomegalovirus. SCIENCE 192:1134-1137.

Giraldo, G., Beth, E., Haguenau, F., 1972. Herpes type virus particles in tissue culture of Kaposi sarcoma from different geographic regions. JNCI 49:1509-1526.

Giraldo, G., Beth, E., Kourilsky, F.M., et al., 1975. Antibody patterns to herpes virus in kaposi's sarcoma: Association of European kaposi's sarcoma with cytomegalovirus. INT. J. CANCER 15:839-848.

Giraldo, G., Beth, L., Henle, W., 1978. Antibody patterns to herpes virus in kaposi's sarcoma: Serological associates of American Kaposi's sarcoma with cytomegalovirus. INT. J. CANCER 72:126-131.

Giraldo, G., Beth, E., Huang, E. S. 1980. Kaposi's sarcoma and its relationships to cytomegalovirus (CMV) III CNV, DNA, and CMV early antigens in Kaposi's sarcoma. INTERNATIONAL J. OF CANCER 26(1):23-29.

Giraldo, G. et al., 1981. Etiological implications on Kaposi's sarcoma. ANTIBIOTICS AND CHEMO-THERAPY 29:580-581.

Lang, D. J., Kummer, J. F., Hartly, D. P., 1975. Cytomegalovirus in semen: Observations in selected populations. THE J. OF INFECTIOUS DISEASES 132:472-473.

May, A. G., Betts, R. F., Andrus, C. C., et al., 1982. Effect of Cytomegalovirus on renal transplantation.

NEW YORK STATE J. OF MED. July 1982:1199-1206.

Meyers, J. D., Flournoy, N., and Thomas, E. D., 1980. Cytomegalovirus infection and specific cell-mediated immunity after bone marrow transplantation. J. INFECT. DISEASES 142:816-824.

Pass, R. F. August, Anna M., et al., 1982. Cytomegalovirus infection in a day-care center. NEW ENGLAND J. MED. 307(8):477-479 (Aug. 19).

Quinnan, Gerald V., Kirmani, N., Rook, A. H., et al. 1982. Cytotoxic T cells in cytomegalovirus infection: HLA-restricted T-lymphocyte and non-T-lymphocyte cytotoxic responses correlate with recovery from cytomegalovirus infection in bone-marrow-transplant recipients. NEW ENGL. J. MED. 307:7-13.

Rinaldo, Charles R., et al. 1980. Mechanisms of immunosuppression in cytomegalovirus mononucleosis. THE J. OF INFECTIOUS DISEASES 141:488-495.

Sordillo, P., Markovich, R., and Hardy, W., 1982. Search for evidence of feline leukemia virus infection in humans with leukemias, lymphomas or soft tissue sarcomas. JNCI 69:333-337.

Spiers A., and Robbins, C., 1982. Cytomegalovirus infection simulating lymphoma in a homosexual man. LANCET I(8283):1248-1249 May 29.

Snydman, D. R., Rudders, R. A. Daoust, P., et al. 1982. Infectious mononucleosis in an adult progressing to fatal immunoblastic lymphoma. ANNALS OF INTERNAL MED. 96(ptl):737-742.

Walker, D. J. and Chesney, T., 1982. Cytomegalovirus infection of the skin. THE AM J. DERMATOL. 4(3):263-265.

Idiopathic Autoimmune Thrombocytopenic Purpura

Barriere, H., Bureau, B., and Planchon, B., 1981. Purpura par sensibilisation au (8 MOP) au cours d'uhe puvatherapie. NOUVELLE PRESSE MED. 10(5):337.

Branda, R. F., McCullough, J. J., Tate, D. Y. and Jacobs, H. S. 1978. Plasma exchange in the treatment of fulminant idiopathic (autoimmune)thrombocytopenic purpura. LANCET I (8066):688.

———————, Moldow, C. F., McCullough, J. J. and Jacob, H. S. 1975. Plasma exchange in the treatment of immune disease. TRANSFUSION 1975(15):570.

Bukowski, R. M., Hewlett, J. S., Harris, J. W., et al. 1976. Exchange transfusions in the treatment of thrombtic thrombocytopenic purpura. SEMIN. HEMATOL 1976(13):219.

Claas, Frans, Runia-van-Nieuwkoop, R., van den Berge, W., and van Rood, J. J. 1982. Interaction of penicillin with HLA-A and B antigens. HUMAN IMMUNOLOGY 5:83-90 Penicillin-induced ITP.

Fitchen, J. J., Cline, M. J., Saxon, A., Golde, D. W. 1979. Serum inhibitors of hematopoiesis in a patient with aplastic anemia and systemic lupus erythematosus. Recovery after exchange plasmapheresis. AM. J. MED. 66(3):537.

Hymes, K. B., Shulman, S., et al., 1979. A solid-phase radioimmunoassay for bound anti-platelet antibody: studies on 45 patients with autoimmune platelet disorders. JOURNAL OF LABORATORY AND CLINICAL MEDICINE 94:639-648.

Imbach, P., d'Apuzzo, V., Hirt, A., et al., 1981. High-dose intravenous gammaglobulin for idiopathic thrombocytopenic purpura in childhood. LANCET I(8232):1228-1230.

Johnson, J. P., Whitman, W., Briggs, W. A., and Wilson, C. B. 1978. Plasmapheresis and immunosuppressive agents in antibasement membrane antibody-induced Goodpasture's syndrome. AM. J. MED. 64(2):354.

Kelton, John G., 1981. Vaccination associated relapse of immune thrombocytpenia. JAMA 245(4):

Lackner, H. L., Karpatkin, S., 1975. Association of anti-platelet antibody with functional platelet disorders. AM. J. MED 59:599.

Lockwood, C. M., Rees, A. J., Pearson, T. A., et al. 1976. Immunosuppression and plasma exchange in the treatment of Goodpasture's syndrome. LANCET I (7962):711.

Lurhuma, A. Z., Riccome, H., and Masson, P. L. 1977. The occurrence of circulating immune complexes and viral antigens in idiopathic thrombocytopenic purpura. CLIN. EXP. IMMUNOL. 1977(78):49.

Marder, V. J., Nusbacher, J., and Anderson, F. W. 1981. One-year follow-up of Plasma Exchange therapy in 14 patients with idiopathic thrombocytopenic purpura. TRANSFUSION 21(3):291-298.

Minchinton, R. M., Waters, A. H., Malpas, J. S., et al., 1982. Autoimmune thrombocytopenia after autologous bone-marrow transplantation. LANCET II (8294):391.

Morris, L., Distenfeld, A., Amorosi, E., Karpatkin, S., 1982. Autoimmune thrombocytopenic purpura in homosexual men. ANN. INT. MED. 96(pt 1):714-717.

Morris, L. B., et al., 1982. Increased apparent autoimmune thrombocytopenic purpura (ATP) in homosexual men. CLINICAL RESEARCH 30(2):A324.

Nenci, Giusepe, et al., 1981. Infustion of vincristine-loaded platelets in Acute ITP refractory to steroids: An alternative to Splenectomy. ACTA HEMATOL. 66:117-121.

Schmidt, R. E., Budde, U., Schafer, G., and Stroehmann, I. 1981. High-Dose intravenous gammaglobulin for idiopathic thrombocytopenic purpura. LANCET II (8244):475-476.

Verrier, Jones J., Cumming, R. H., Bucnall, R., et al. 1976. Plasmapheresis in the management of acute systemic lupus erythematosis. LANCET I(7962):709.

Zindberg, Morton, Francus, T., Weksler, M., et al., 1982. Abnormal autologous mixed lymphocyte reaction in autoimmune thrombocytopenic purpura. BLOOD 59(1):148-151.

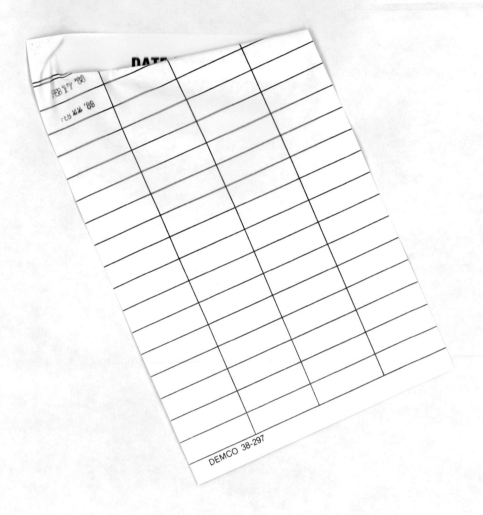